# Praise for *Kava*

"A must-read for anyone interested in conquering stress.
Kava is Nature's answer for anxiety."
**–Dharma Singh Khalsa, M.D., author of *Brain Longevity***

"This dynamic team of authors presents a practical guide to
understanding and using a remarkable herb to ameliorate the
effects of our stressful lives."
**–Janet Zand, N.D., L.Ac., O.M.D.,
cofounder and formulator of ZAND Herbal Formulas,
author of *Smart Medicine for a Healthier Child***

"What a pleasure it is to finally have an answer to an often-asked
question, 'What is Kava?' Here is the complete story of this remarkable plant, from its historic origins to its present-day use,
told accurately and entertainingly in a single reference source."
**–Alexander Shulgin, Ph.D., author of *PIHKAL* and *TIHKAL***

Kava quiets the mind;
the world gains no new color or rose tint;
it fits in its place and in one easily understandable whole.

—*E. M. Lemert (1967)*

# KAVA

## Nature's Answer to Stress, Anxiety, and Insomnia

**HYLA CASS, M.D., AND**
**TERRENCE McNALLY**

**PRIMA HEALTH**

A Division of Prima Publishing

*To the spirit of kava,*
*and to the islanders who*
*discovered, cultivated, and preserved it*
*over centuries.*

**Warning—Disclaimer**

This book is not intended to provide medical advice and is sold with the understanding that the publisher and the author are not liable for the misconception or misuse of information provided. The author and Prima Publishing shall have neither liability nor responsibility to any person or entity with respect to any loss, damage, or injury caused or alleged to be caused directly or indirectly by the information contained in this book or the use of any products mentioned. Readers should not use any of the products discussed in this book without the advice of a medical professional.

The production of this work was not underwritten in any way by the pharmaceutical companies whose products are mentioned.

**Library of Congress Cataloging-in-Publication Data**

Cass, Hyla.
  Kava : nature's answer to stress, anxiety, and insomnia / Hyla Cass, and Terrence McNally
      p.   cm.
  Includes bibliographical references and index.
  ISBN 0-7615-1667-0
  1. Kava plant—Therapeutic use. 2. Kava (Beverage)—Therapeutic use.
  I. McNally, Terrence. II. Title.
  RM666.K6C37   1998
615'.32325—dc21                                                                98-25977
                                                                                      CIP

98 99 00 01 HH 10 9 8 7 6 5 4 3 2 1
Printed in the United States of America

# CONTENTS

*Acknowledgments*   vii

*Introduction*   xi

**1**  Kava: The Route Ahead   1

**2**  Stress and Anxiety   11

**3**  Stress and Disease: The Mind–Body Continuum   29

**4**  Anxiety: Psychological Factors   41

**5**  Medications: The Antidepressants and Tranquilizers   53

**6**  What Is Kava?   67

**7**  Chemistry and Actions   81

**8**  Clinical Uses of Kava   91

**9**  Sleep and Insomnia   111

**10**  How to Take Kava   133

**11**  Safety and Contraindications   141

**12**  Herbal Combinations   155

**13**  Diet and Supplements   171

**14**  Managing Stress    191

**15**  Listening to Kava:
The High Road from Doing to Being    205

**16**  Growing Kava    217

**17**  The Economics and Regulation of Kava    229

**18**  Closing Thoughts    243

*Appendix A: Recommended Reading*    251

*Appendix B: Resources*    253

*Appendix C: Kava Beverage Preparation Recipe*    257

*Notes*    258

*Index*    267

# ACKNOWLEDGMENTS

## From Both of Us

Many thanks to Steven Bratman, M.D., medical director for the Prima Health Division, who, during a chance conversation, immediately recognized the importance of this topic, introduced us to Acquisitions Editor Susan Silva, and set things in motion. Steven provided invaluable feedback throughout the writing process, based on his rich knowledge and experience in both natural and conventional medicine. His warmth, writing talent, and clear and gentle guidance when we were "off"—as well as his enthusiasm when we were "right on"—were exceptional and much appreciated.

Susan was always supportive, understanding, and respectful. She handed us over to Michelle McCormack, our project editor, whose dedication helped make our job easier. Michelle was there day and night, even on weekends, to see that the book turned out the way we all envisioned it. And finally, Publicity & Marketing Manager, Robin Lockwood got on the job immediately, enthusiastically, and with complete professionalism.

There is a committed team at Prima—led by President and Founder Ben Dominitz—who have been extraordinarily helpful, professional, and supportive. With a sense of partnership and participation, they have allowed us choices along the way that demonstrate both their integrity and their respect for us as authors.

We sincerely appreciate the intelligence, enthusiasm, and hard work of Zack Stentz, our absurdly overqualified research assistant.

Many others contributed to making this book possible, and we will likely leave out some (either inadvertently or because the list would be too long), but we thank them along with the following: Muggenberg Extracts and their representatives, Jack Klein and Gregory Bonifilio, who generously shared their research material in a readily accessible form. Joerg Gruenwald of Phytopharm Consulting, Berlin, for his valuable insight and his understanding of the nuances of German research as it translates into English language and American culture. For their wisdom, knowledge, analysis, and humor, we thank Mark Blumenthal of the American Botanical Council; Jerry Cott of the National Institute of Mental Health; Ed Smith of HerbPharm; Rob McCaleb of Herb Research Foundation; Chris Kilham, author and herbal consultant (Cowboy Marketing); Loren Israelsen of LDI Group; Peggy and Bill Brevoort of East Earth Herb; Floyd Leaders of Botanical Enterprises; Bettina Soholm of ESCOP; Steven Dentali of Natural Products Consulting Services; Terry Willard of Wild Rose College of Natural Healing; Don Brown of *Natural Products Research Consultants;* Michael McGuffin of McZand Herbal; Christopher Hobbs, herbalist and author; Raleigh Pinsky, author of *101 Ways to Promote Yourself;* Roy Upton of The American Herbal Pharmacopeia; and Gary Friedman of Cosmopolitan Trading (Kaviar), who was always available with valuable, first-hand information.

We thank our friends who have inspired, advised, and above all, believed in us: Ann and Sasha Shulgin, Jim Autry, Jim Strohecker, Mark Litwak, Carlos Warter, and Andrew Weil (who agreed with us that kava was "next").

# From Hyla

I thank my loving and supportive family: My late father, Dr. Isadore Cass, who was my inspiration as a physician; my dear mother, Miriam Cass; my daughter, Alison; and my sisters, Sharon, Judy, and Elaine.

I could not have written this book without Debby Stover, my loving, talented, and conscientious assistant who kept my office in order and the world at bay. I am immensely grateful to the members of my alternative medicine support group, who have taught me much of what I know. They continue to educate and inspire me, as well as each other, and they are also my dear friends. Drs. Michael Rosenbaum, Murray Susser, Cynthia Watson, Mel Werbach, and Janet Zand were especially helpful with this book.

Lastly, I want to thank Terrence for his spirit of adventure, immense knowledge about everything, quickness in grasping new information, ability to see the larger picture and organize it for me, writing talent, patience, support, affection, and wild sense of humor.

# From Terrence

I am deeply grateful to my parents, Edward and Marcella McNally; my siblings, Marcella, Brian, Michael, Edward, and Suzanne; and my two 98-year-old grandmothers, Claire and Yvonne, for being there for me without fail.

Thanks to all those with whom I've shared writing and exploration over the years, including Sara Davidson, Michael Schiffer, Michael Catlin, and Steve Bornstein; to radio station KPFK for giving me the opportunity to learn from my wise and committed guests; to all those who have indulged and sharpened my generalist's mind over the years;

to those who keep the hope of natural and holistic systems alive in the world; and to my oldest friend, the late Jonathan Waxman, who invited me to freely share his home (Hawaii) and gave me the gift of its living spirit. Lastly, I want to thank Hyla for inviting me to discover kava and write this book with her. Her curiosity, friendship, patience, stamina, and willingness to let the work be the boss are inspiring. Her confidence in me will be forever appreciated.

# INTRODUCTION

We, the authors, would like to share with you some of the background of this book. First, we wish to acknowledge each other, Terrence and Hyla, for following our instincts and excitement about a little-known herb that piqued our curiosity and led us on a mutual adventure of discovery and creativity. Writing a book together presents many challenges—and we met them all with mutual respect, graciousness, and appreciation for the gifts we each brought to the process (most of the time, anyway). We both attended conferences, gathered research, conducted interviews, analyzed material, and wrote together and separately, often not knowing afterward which of us had written a specific passage.

In terms of author's voice, "we" is used most of the time throughout *Kava*. When we use "I", although we generally do not specify who is speaking, the context should make it clear. All the clinical material is based on Hyla's professional experience. She takes the lead with regard to medicine and the presentation and analysis of research, while Terrence does so with regard to history, economics, and other social sciences.

In May 1997, the wisest and luckiest thing we did was attend the First International Botanical Symposium on Kava and other Medicinal Plants of the South Pacific, in Kona, Hawaii. We'd been considering writing this book for several months and decided to jump-start the process by thus immersing ourselves in the world of kava. By doing this, we experienced a critical moment in the evolution of a cultural, commercial, and medical phenomenon. The few days we spent in Kona transformed our creative journey, as well as the task itself. The book could no longer simply be a report about the clinical value of a newly popular substance. We had become participants, exploring from multiple angles a subject, kava, that has been in constant and accelerating motion ever since.

One could probably write a perfectly good book about kava without actually experiencing how the herb is held and used very differently in different countries and cultures. Yet we were able to do that first hand in Kona. During a day-long field trip to a Hawaiian kava plantation, for example, we had the good fortune to spend time with an American representative of a German manufacturer, an esteemed ethnobotanist, a Canadian herbalist, and a Tongan agricultural development official.

Evenings were spent tasting various brands and "cultivars" of kava. As with fine wines, kava is an acquired taste, and we acquired it in Kona. We also developed a vital interest in getting to know this herb—not *about* it, but actually "taking it in." Lastly, we cultivated a circle of friends within the kava "community," with whom we've shared freshly extracted kava ("island style") several times over the course of the past year. Many of these people were mentioned in our acknowledgements, as all of them deserve to be.

We feel a sense of responsibility to the islanders who cultivated kava for centuries, to the many players working to bring kava's gifts to the wider global population, to those who stand to benefit, and to the herb itself. We have told kava's story to the best of our abilities, well aware that we have been aiming at a moving target. We offer this book to readers with the knowledge that kava's story continues to be written.

We wish we had more time, but that is the nature of publishing. That's what deadlines (and publishers) are for. There is always more to say, more refinement of what has been said, and probably things we wish we'd never said (we may deny them later, or blame the editor). Often, when the intensity got too high or we were totally exhausted, Terrence would say something absurdly funny, and we'd burst out laughing. This comic relief broke the tension, helping to shift our perspectives and restore our energy. We also took a lot of kava. Believe me, it helped us handle the stress and tension. In this book, we claim kava does that without dulling mental sharpness. You be the judge.

## CHAPTER 1

# Kava:
# The Route Ahead

Kava, an herb used ceremonially for centuries in the islands of the South Pacific, has the remarkable ability to promote relaxation without affecting mental sharpness, making it the perfect natural supplement for today's frantic, stress-filled lifestyle. Easing anxiety by creating a sense of peacefulness and oneness between mind and body, kava's soothing effects seem to mirror the laid-back image of the tropical culture. Safe, free of side effects, and non-addictive, kava is not only calming, but has been shown to actually *enhance* perception, awareness, and clarity of thought.

## Sharing Kava

We are at the First International Botanical Symposium on Kava on the Big Island of Hawaii. This is one conference that isn't being held in Kona for the golf. Participants from all over the United States, Germany, Holland, Paris, Tonga, Samoa, and Fiji have come to Hawaii because kava grows here. Kava—the plant, the beverage, and its ceremonial and social culture—is a central part of life in most islands of the Pacific. In a poetic bit of botany, the herb seems to carry the essence of the islands in its roots. Modern research confirms that it is effective for the treatment of anxiety, and unlike most other stress relievers, it actually enhances concentration and memory.

It is spring 1997, and the conference has attracted scientists, doctors, writers, suppliers—everyone from native island growers to European representatives of the world's biggest distributors. On a point overlooking the ocean, the setting is spectacular. Waterfalls spill over lava rocks throughout the gardens where lush greens mix with the brilliant reds and yellows of exotic plants. We empty out of a darkened auditorium into the golden light of late afternoon and shuffle onto straw mats laid out in a circle for us to sit on.

Six young Hawaiian men in pale yellow sarongs kneel in the center chanting. One man, who looks to be the oldest, sits in saffron, kneading a mush of ground kava root in a large wooden bowl. At a signal, the chanting stops, and the elder intones a blessing. One of the younger men approaches the bowl and kneels facing the leader, who hands him a coconut shell filled with kava. He raises the shell above his head with both hands, rises, and with head bowed and knees well apart, walks through the crowd, then turns behind a couple of palm trees and pours the kava to the ground as a libation to the gods. He returns to his position up front. In succession, each of the other men comes forward as the first. The kava maker squeezes some of the liquid through a strainer into a shell, and one by one, each accepts the shell, turns around on bent knees, walks hunched over for a few steps, then straightens. The first moves to one of the organizers of the symposium and presents the shell. He accepts the shell with both hands and holds it aloft briefly, observing the sacred nature of the moment. He then takes it to his lips and drinks the contents in one gulp. The natives and several of the attendees clap three times.

The bearer takes back the shell, returns to the bowl, and the other servers proceed in the same way to offer the drink to a dozen or so members of the crowd. Then they stop serving, rise, and dance, singing a rousing, aggressive chant, each in turn taking the lead. When the last finishes, the elder says "mahalo" ("thank you" in Hawaiian). In silence they pick up their implements and walk past us across the green lawn toward the sea.

We were among the lucky ones to be introduced to kava in this way. The liquid was lukewarm, watery, and a bit muddy, with a bitter taste. Within seconds it began to numb my tongue and the inside of my mouth. Over the next few minutes, as we all walked to the beach to take in a majestic pacific sunset, my whole body relaxed. The effect was gradual, like soft waves washing over me. My neck moved freely, and my knees, which were a little sore after kneeling on the mats, loosened. The sunset needed no help, but sights and sounds became a bit sharper and more vivid. The overall subtlety of the experience is worth emphasizing. Though my senses were heightened, my mind was clear, and I was in absolute control of my faculties. My face felt softened, and I'm sure I had the slightest silly smile. All was well with the world.

Similar scenes have taken place throughout the islands of the South Pacific for centuries. This peaceful plant is also drunk informally on a regular basis, when villagers gather to unwind and share stories after a hard day's work.

At the end of a work day half a world away, on congested city streets and freeways, a very different scene unfolds. You sit behind the wheel, stuck in traffic, feeling frustrated by another situation that you cannot control. You left the office a little late; you have to pick your kids up from soccer and get the dog from the vet before they close. You still haven't figured out what's for dinner or how you're going to get your sales reports done by tomorrow. You glance at the guy in the car next to you, recognizing his tight and weary expression as your own.

# Stress: A National Epidemic

You are not alone. More and more Americans live much of their time in a constant state of anxiety, battling stress at every turn—leading to fatigue, depression, burnout, physical illness, and death. A modern office worker afraid of being chewed out by the boss experiences many of the same physiological events as a caveman 50,000 years ago about to be chewed *on* by a saber-toothed tiger. The "fight or flight" response—that complex set of physical and psychological responses we call stress—erupts spontaneously in a human body mobilized for danger.

"Epidemic" is not too strong a word to describe the rates of stress we are currently seeing in the United States. A Gallup poll reports that up to 25% of the American work force suffers from excess stress or anxiety. Fifteen percent of the U.S. population has had an anxiety disorder, and one in five Americans suffer from stress-related insomnia.[1, 2, 3] We all experience stress. Any alteration in a person's environment can cause it, including changes related to work, finances, relationships, or lifestyle. It can be brought about by something as simple as standing in a slow-moving line.

This book includes self-administered questionnaires that allow you to assess the number and severity of stressors to which you are currently exposed, as well as the number and intensity of anxiety symptoms you may be experiencing as a result.

Our bodies pay a price for years of stress. Sixty percent of doctor visits are connected to stress and the physical ailments it can cause. The cost to business is $50 to $75 billion a year. Modern research shows that stress can be fatal, and may be an underlying cause of our most pernicious diseases—heart disease, high blood pressure, arthritis, and cancer.

# A Vicious Cycle

Together, fear, stress, and anxiety engender a truly vicious cycle, which feeds on itself, reducing our vitality. Just as the caveman could see only two options—fight or flight—the chronic stress that pervades our lives limits our vision in every way, narrowing our view of what's possible in our jobs, our relationships, and our society. If a cornered animal is dangerous to himself as well as to others, how much more before an entire society that feels that way?

Too many of us believe that we can't afford to give up our stress level for fear that we will lose our "edge." We put off relaxing until we complete the next project, contract, or term paper. However, research shows that a state of relaxed alertness allows us to work better and smarter. True health involves both mind and body. The workaholic style, based on pushing ourselves "just a little harder," is not the answer. The mind may be willing, but the body will collapse under the load.

In grappling with the complex problems of stress and anxiety, conventional medicine usually relies on the prescription of powerful psychoactive drugs. The drawbacks of this approach include the potential for addiction, mental and physical impairment, and the serious health risks that accompany their use. Also, by focusing exclusively on treating the symptoms, chemical treatment by itself fails to address the underlying issues and problems that cause stress in the first place. We will discuss the problems and side effects of specific drugs later in the book, comparing and contrasting them with their natural and herbal counterparts.

Psychotherapy is also often used in the conventional treatment of stress. While this may not solve the external causes, the process helps us to uncover the factors in our own psyche that allow stress to thrive, and to develop internal and external strategies for stress reduction. In a Catch-22, however, anxiety often interferes with learning, thus sabotaging the therapy process. Have you ever tried to memorize some material just before an exam, and felt you were staring at total gibberish? Not only is a depleted mind unable to think clearly, a burned out body-mind lacks the energy to make the changes necessary to improve the situation.

## Nature's Answers

We believe a variety of natural therapies, used singly or in combination with each other, can prove extremely useful in managing this epidemic of the 1990s. Safe, natural, and inexpensive, kava may have a particular contribution to make. Research has demonstrated its capacity to promote relaxation without a loss in mental sharpness. One could say kava has the ability "to wake you up as it calms you down."

Increasing productivity while reducing anxiety is probably a dream of 90% of the people in 90% of the skyscrapers in 90% of the cities in the world. It is easy to joke that kava has been wasted on South Sea islanders. After all, what do they know from stress? Hong Kong and Manhattan are the kinds of islands that need kava.

The media and the public are suddenly "discovering" remedies that have proven effective for centuries in traditional use, and for twenty years in my own clinical experience. When St. John's wort, an herbal remedy for depression, was the subject of a cover story in *Newsweek* and a prominent feature on television's *20/20*, its use increased by 1,000. The subsequent success of my book, *St. John's Wort: Nature's Blues Buster*, was one more indication to me that people are hungry for practical information about the use of natural remedies for depression.

We recognize, however, that there is an equal, if not greater, demand for information on natural treatments for the tension and anxiety that affect nearly everyone. In this time of unprecedented uncertainty and accelerating change, we want to introduce kava as an effective component of a holistic approach to mental and emotional health.

## Let Go of Tension and Anxiety with Kava

Kava is already commonly prescribed in Europe, and scientific research suggests that it is as effective as Valium-type relaxants (benzodiazepines) in treating anxiety, but without their sedative effects. One German study of patients diagnosed with anxiety syndrome found that the participants experienced dramatic improvements after just one week of kava use.[4] Kava doesn't cause addiction, habituation, or side effects; is not expensive; and is available without a prescription. Tests have also indicated that kava, while relaxing both muscles and emotions, actually sharpens concentration and memory.

In addition, kava works socially as well as individually. Our society, for the most part, deals with problems on an individual basis: "It's your problem"—your personality, bad habits, childhood traumas, brain chemistry, or diet. Though there are exceptions—such as 12-step recovery programs (modeled after Alcoholics Anonymous) and couples or family therapy—we have all but abandoned traditions of extended family, and religious or tribal experiences that could provide comfort and support in our lives. Throughout the islands of the South Pacific, kava's long history of communal use has served to foster connection, communication, and even conflict resolution. Clinical experience has shown that it promotes similar effects in modern settings.

In this book you will learn how to use kava. We will answer questions regarding the best forms to take it in, recommended dosages, matters of safety, and the various combinations with other healing and fortifying nutrients. We will also discuss briefly how it works, including its chemistry and pharmacology. In addition, we will tell you about some of kava's colorful history, and introduce you to the complex issues of politics, economics, and government regulation that may impact its development as a mainstream supplement in the United States and internationally.

We discuss kava and other natural supplements in the wider context of the revolution in health care now taking place in the United States. Faced with soaring costs, the frustrations of managed care, and the failure of modern medicine to provide adequate solutions to critical health problems, Americans are seeking alternative solutions in ever-increasing numbers.

In a 1998 study, conducted by John Astin at Stanford and published in the *Journal of the American Medical Association* (JAMA), 40% of respondents had used some form of alternative health care during the preceding year. This is up from 33% in the often-cited Eisenberg/Harvard study published in the *New England Journal of Medicine* in 1993. Moreover, in the 1998 study, anxiety was tied at 31% for the second most frequently cited health problem treated with alternative therapies.[5]

With kava as part of a natural approach to stress, we may begin to replace anxiety and inertia with flow and momentum. When we are less at war with ourselves and each other, we can make healthier choices in all areas of our lives. The most important benefit of kava may well be that as we break the stress cycle, we will have the energy and ability to integrate new life changes—something that is difficult, if not impossible, to do until we can get off the stress treadmill. In this book, we suggest that kava may be one of nature's unique keys with which to unlock the door to healthier living in a mad, mad world.

# Not By Kava Alone

At the same time, let us make clear that kava by itself is not enough. In addition to its internal synergy, kava, like many other herbs, is often particularly useful in combination with other nutrients. This book will describe specific formulas for particular conditions. For example, someone troubled by insomnia would take kava with valerian, another relaxing herb. A student in a frantic push during finals might take kava and ginseng; kava to relax and focus and ginseng to restore both mental and physical energy.

While we believe kava offers a natural means to reduce the costs of the stressful lives we lead, we can't help but feel that the message of kava is more than that. Within its age-old social context, the drinking of kava takes place in a "community" of people who share the release of tension and anxiety, and move together into an experience of greater well-being and sociability. Earlier this century, Tom Harrisson wrote in *Savage Civilization,* "You feel friendly . . . never cross. . . . You cannot hate with kava in you."[6] In this book, we offer you information about the relief available through kava extracts in capsules and tinctures. We also offer you a vision of the world from which it comes.

Finally, confronting many of the self-destructive biases of our frantic workaholic culture, we will make a convincing and welcome case for the intrinsic value of mindfulness, calmness, and pleasure. The combination of all of the above, from herbs to diet, and exercise to specific anti-stress techniques, can lead the reader out of the stress trap and into a more relaxed, healthy, and fulfilling lifestyle.

In kava, we may have not only a significant breakthough in the treatment of stress, anxiety, and insomnia, but a possible bridge to new ways of being. Kava can facilitate the shift from the old model of conflict and domination (which is fear-based) to one of partnership and cooperation (based on trust and respect).

In the next chapters, we will present the psychological roots of these problems and their conventional solutions, followed by a return to older, more natural approaches, based on tradition and backed by research.

## CHAPTER 2

# Stress and Anxiety

People are frayed by the inescapable pressure of technology. . . .
They feel caged by their jobs even as they put in more overtime.

*—Newsweek*

## Stone-Age Stress

Contrary to what we may think, stress is not a twentieth century invention. It has been with us since the dawn of human
existence. Imagine Nog, a prehistoric man, venturing out of
his cave in his daily search for food. Feeling calm, enjoying
the moment, he breathes in the cool air. A sense of well-
being envelops him as he takes in the scenery around him.
Suddenly his serenity is broken by a crashing in the forest
nearby. Nog's whole body instantly shifts from a state of relaxation to one of tension, his heart pounding, his muscles

taut. As the rustling in the woods slows and moves closer, his mouth becomes dry, and a cold shiver shoots down his spine. He looks around, grabs a sharp piece of rock, and stands awaiting the enemy. With little thought, his body instinctively prepares to either fight or flee.

Several steps in front of him, the enemy emerges from thick undergrowth. A panting mountain lion takes a quick look at the caveman, then just as quickly turns and disappears again among the trees. Though the caveman's senses remain alert, his breathing eases, and he returns swiftly to the cave. He will rest, leaving his outing for later. There are no clocks or deadlines here, only his ongoing physical need to stay alive. He has survived this round, with no apparent after-effects. He is not likely to stay awake tonight mulling over this recent escape or worrying incessantly about it happening again.

Nog is once again in harmony with his surroundings. Without a great deal of analysis or anticipation, he relies on his built-in emergency response for survival. The mountain lion does the same. Nog's reaction may remind you of your pet cat, who can curl up and fall asleep minutes after narrowly escaping the wheels of a speeding automobile.

## Contemporary Distress

Compare Nog's encounter with the scenario of a twentieth century urban man, Ned. Battling traffic to arrive at the office twenty minutes late, he's greeted by an alarming memo from his boss. A client is threatening to kill an important deal, and Ned's promotion could be in danger. His heart pounds and his muscles become taut as anxiety escalates to true tension. His mouth is dry, his head aches, and a shiver runs down his spine. His metal paperweight suddenly attracts his attention, and he resists the primitive impulse to bash someone over the head with it—but who would he bash? The boss? The client? The rival? Instead he smashes his fist down hard on his desk, hurting himself in the process. Then, in pain and resignation, he reaches into his desk drawer for an aspirin—or a Valium.

Ned no longer has to grapple with the dangers of the wild. But the instinct for "fight or flight" is very much present in the concrete jungle in which he now lives. Seemingly endless hours of work at an insecure job, sandwiched between a lengthy commute, contribute to the phenomenon we call stress. Unlike his jungle ancestor, he cannot physically escape his situation, nor does he feel able to let go of worry and fear. Danger in one form or another is constant. To all the threats in his environment, he adds those in his mind, with memories of the past and fear for the future.

## The Survival of Stress, the Stress of Survival

Evolution moves slowly. Biological traits can linger in a species long after the original reason for their development has disappeared. California ground squirrels display stereotypical rattlesnake-response behavior—throwing dirt and fluffing up their tails, even in regions where rattlesnakes have been extinct for 70,000 to 300,000 years. North American pronghorn antelopes can achieve speeds of 60 miles an hour, though any North American predator capable of running that fast has been extinct for 10,000 years or more.[1] Our bodies respond to stress as if we were still in the jungle. We are increasingly alarmed by an overstimulating environment of our own making that provides inadequate opportunities for release.

Perhaps only in the last several decades has this become dangerous. Just when advances in hygiene and the use of antibiotics greatly improved our chances for longevity, we began to pay a steep price for other aspects of progress, in the form of stress-related diseases. In the mid-1930s, physiologist Walter Cannon, who first named the "fight or flight" response, pointed out a shift in what ailed Americans. ". . . Serious infections, formerly extensive and disastrous, have markedly decreased or almost disappeared . . . meanwhile conditions involving strain in the nervous system have been greatly augmented."[2] As we shall see, we have new conditions now that Cannon never even dreamed of.

# Defining Terms

The word "stress" means different things to different people. Some think of it as tension, others view it as anxiety. The best definition we have found is the following: "Stress is the inability to cope with a real, perceived, or imagined threat to one's mental, physical, emotional or spiritual well-being which results in a series of physiological responses and adaptations."[3] It includes changes in perception, emotions, behavior, and physical functioning. Short-term stress will not usually cause any long-term problems. However, prolonged, continuous stress will cause long-term problems. It suppresses the immune system and depletes the body of essential nutrients. Trivial everyday problems suddenly become unmanageable and exaggerated beyond all proportion. The person may feel tense, moody, and hyperactive. But in the long-term, the damage is potentially much more serious. For example, high blood pressure, elevated cholesterol levels, and heart disease are all stress-induced diseases.

### Risk Assessment

A wide variety of personal crises and events can produce stress. We usually consider stress to be the result of negative experiences—job loss, ill health, or marital conflict, for example. However, there is also stress associated with positive change. Human beings tend to be creatures of habit. Thus, drastic changes in routine, even if positive—such as a new marriage, or going on a much-anticipated trip—can be highly stressful.

The Social Readjustment Rating Scale, developed by Holmes and Rahe in 1967, is a tool often used by physicians and therapists to rate stress levels. The scale displays a wide variety of stressors, such as loss of employment, a death in the family, and struggling to pay a mortgage, and rates each according to its stress-causing potential. The following scale, adapted from the classic by Holmes and Rahe, lists these stresses and allows you to score yourself on your own "risk potential" scale.

Go through the following list, and circle any event that has affected you in the last twelve months. Then add up the total mean values.

### Holmes-Rahe Stressor Scale

| Rank | Life Event | Mean Value |
|------|-----------|------------|
| 1 | Death of spouse | 100 |
| 2 | Divorce | 73 |
| 3 | Marital separation | 65 |
| 4 | Jail term | 63 |
| 5 | Death of close family member | 63 |
| 6 | Personal injury or illness | 53 |
| 7 | Marriage | 50 |
| 8 | Fired from job | 47 |
| 9 | Marital reconciliation | 45 |
| 10 | Retirement | 45 |
| 11 | Change in health of family member | 44 |
| 12 | Pregnancy | 40 |
| 13 | Sex difficulties | 39 |

*(continued)*

## Holmes-Rahe Stressor Scale *(continued)*

| Rank | Life Event | Mean Value |
|------|-----------|-----------|
| 14 | Gain of new family member | 39 |
| 15 | Business adjustment | 39 |
| 16 | Change in financial status | 38 |
| 17 | Death of close friend | 37 |
| 18 | Change to different line of work | 36 |
| 19 | Change in number of arguments with spouse | 35 |
| 20 | Large mortgage | 31 |
| 21 | Foreclosure of mortgage or loan | 30 |
| 22 | Change in responsibilities at work | 29 |
| 23 | Son or daughter leaving home | 29 |
| 24 | Trouble with in-laws | 29 |
| 25 | Outstanding personal achievement | 28 |
| 26 | Spouse begins or stops work | 26 |
| 27 | Begin or end school | 26 |
| 28 | Change in living conditions | 25 |
| 29 | Revision of personal habits | 24 |
| 30 | Trouble with boss | 23 |
| 31 | Change in work hours or conditions | 20 |
| 32 | Change in residence | 20 |
| 33 | Change in schools | 20 |
| 34 | Change in recreation | 19 |
| 35 | Change in church activities | 19 |
| 36 | Change in social activities | 18 |
| 37 | Small mortgage | 17 |
| 38 | Change in sleeping habits | 16 |
| 39 | Change in number of family get-togethers | 15 |
| 40 | Change in eating habits | 15 |
| 41 | Vacation | 13 |

### Holmes-Rahe Stressor Scale

| Rank | Life Event | Mean Value |
|------|------------|------------|
| 42 | Christmas | 12 |
| 43 | Minor violations of the law | 11 |
| | **Total Score** | _____ |

According to Holmes and Rahe, people with scores totaling 300 or more have an 80% chance of developing a major illness or falling into a clinical depression during the following year. Those scoring between 200 and 300 points have a 50% risk of falling victim to illness or depression. And those who rate below 200 points are considered at relatively low risk.[4]

These averages assume that all of us respond in the same way to similar stressors. However, it is not just the amount of stress that counts. Some people manage stress more easily than others. The next questionnaire will let you know how you are doing in this regard.

Following is an explanation of how stress affects your mind and body. Later chapters will tell you how best to handle it, with advice on supplements, diet, lifestyle, and specific coping techniques.

# The Stress Response

Nobel Prize recipient Dr. Hans Selye, the father of stress research, first defined stress as "the nonspecific response of the body to any demand."[5] As is so often true with science, Selye discovered the stress response without really looking for it. In early experiments with hormone chemistry, he tried to isolate the effects of individual hormones on laboratory rats. What he discovered was at first confusing. No matter what hormone was injected, the internal damage it

## Signs of Stress Assessment

Now that you know the potential problem caused by these events, you can evaluate your actual responses. We need a certain amount of stress to keep us motivated. But when stress takes over our lives, it can adversely affect our health. The next step is to recognize some of the signs, as listed below.

*Scoring:* Never = 0; Occasionally = 1;
Often = 2; Always = 3

1. You have difficulty relaxing                    _____

2. You have a persistent feeling of unease         _____

3. You are tense, irritable, or impatient          _____

4. You find it difficult to concentrate or to
   make decisions                                  _____

5. You are frustrated by the incompetence
   of others                                       _____

6. You have a dry mouth and sweaty palms           _____

7. You smoke or drink excessively (especially by
   others' standards)                              _____

8. You feel a lack of interest in sex

caused in the rat was always the same. He purified the chemicals extensively, thinking that some impurity was the cause, and even used combinations of hormones, but it made no difference. The damage was always the same. Three rather dramatic effects occurred within the bodies of all the animals he injected: the adrenal glands became significantly enlarged; the thymus gland, responsible for fighting disease, atrophied; and the animal developed ulcers. Puzzled over why different hormones produced the same

9. You worry about little events of the day and
   are unable to shut your mind off          _____

10. You find it hard to relate to people       _____

11. You are competitive and aggressive in the
    things you do                             _____

12. You take on too much                       _____

13. You take on unrealistic deadlines
    (and worry about not meeting them)         _____

14. You have difficulty delegating             _____

15. You eat quickly                            _____

16. You have aching limbs or recurrent headaches _____

17. You have problems sleeping                 _____

18. You feel burdened financially              _____

*Scores:* 0–15: you are in fine shape, able to roll with the
         punches
       16–26: you are mildly stressed; it's time to reexamine
         your lifestyle
       27–40: you are quite stressed; pay attention to these
         warning signs
       41–54: you are highly stressed; you must take
         measures to reduce your stress level

results, Selye had one of those "Eureka!" experiences of which researchers dream. He realized the experiment was demonstrating that all stress, regardless of origin or type, affects the body the same way. Any challenge to the body's equilibrium will put it into an emergency response mode, which over time, will cause damage. Selye postulated that changes in our environment and life patterns cause corresponding changes in our bodies, such as increased muscle tension and blood pressure. These adaptations are useful in understanding stress. It is evident that inadequate, inappropriate, or exaggerated adaptation can lead to complications.

# Physiology

When we encounter a stressor, our body reacts with a cascade of neuro-hormonal changes. The brain releases CRF (corticotropin releasing factor), which immediately arouses the central nervous system. The *hypothalamus,* a part of the brain that serves as the command center of the endocrine system, sends a signal to the *pituitary gland,* the body's master gland, which lies right beneath the hypothalamus. The pituitary releases multiple hormones, including ACTH (adrenocorticotropic hormone). This signals the *adrenal glands,* which lie on top of the kidneys, to release two hormones, *adrenaline* and *cortisol.* The brain also releases natural painkillers such as endorphins.

This "fight or flight" response allows the body to react to danger. Adrenaline is responsible for obvious physical effects, such as increases in respiration, heart rate, and blood pressure. Cortisol causes the liver to release glucose into the bloodstream for quick energy. To enable the body to use all of its energy reserves in dealing with the emergency at hand, it also depresses the immune system. This originally made sense: Focus all your resources on the immediate external threat. As a result of this rapid deployment, we have more oxygen and sugar available, we push more blood to the brain and muscles, and we are instantly more alert.[6]

As we've seen, the constant complex process of adapting to our environment involves the brain and nervous system; the heart and circulatory system; the liver, spleen, and digestive system; the adrenal glands and immune system; and many other organs. Amazingly sophisticated communication networks function continuously at low levels, monitoring for sudden changes. At times of need, the system surges, preparing us to respond. Individually and collectively, we owe our continued existence to the stress adaptation process.

Selye made some additional distinctions. The environmental changes that set the process in motion he called *stressors*. *Stress* is the normal internal physiological mechanism that adapts us to change. He termed the positive and constructive aspect *eustress,* and he called the negative and destructive aspect *distress*. According to Selye, "Each period of stress, especially if it results from frustrating, unsuccessful struggles, leaves some irreversible chemical scars which accumulate to constitute the signs of tissue aging."[7] Building on the work by Walter Cannon, Selye proposed a three-stage "General Adaptation Syndrome" (GAS). His work demonstrated that mental stress was transmitted into the body's psychosomatic response ("psycho" means mind; "somatic" means body) through the autonomic, endocrine, and immune systems. The GAS consists of alarm, resistance, and finally, exhaustion.

### Phase I: Alarm Reaction

The first response is the alarm reaction, which is caused by certain chemical reactions produced in the brain. These cause the adrenal medulla (or core) to secrete adrenaline and other stress-related hormones. Mobilizing its resources to perform the necessary physical activity, this is the body's first defense mechanism: the "fight or flight" response.

### Phase II: Resistance Reaction

When the body needs to continue its defense mechanism beyond the initial "fight or flight" response, it enters the resistance reaction phase. The adrenal cortex (outer covering) produces hormones called corticosteroids for this resistance reaction. Overuse by the body's defense mechanism in this phase eventually leads to disease.

## *Phase III: Exhaustion*

The autonomic nervous system, endocrine system, and immune system are the three greatest victims of the hormones that the body produces for its initial, but temporary, defense. Once this defense becomes permanent, a chain reaction occurs, impairing the function of all vital organs because of the depletion of all the water-soluble vitamins, including ascorbic acid (vitamin C), the B vitamins, and essential minerals such as magnesium.

The hypothalamus-pituitary-adrenal (HPA) chain of command has served humans well as a means of survival for thousands of years. For those suffering from chronic anxiety and depression, however, this process malfunctions. It appears that continual stress early in life disrupts the cycle. Instead of shutting off once the crisis is over, the process continues, with the hypothalamus continuing to signal the adrenals to produce cortisol. This increased cortisol production exhausts the stress mechanism, leading to fatigue and depression. Cortisol also interferes with serotonin activity, furthering the depressive effect. (For more on serotonin, see Chapter 3.)

Moreover, continually high cortisol levels lead to suppression of the immune system through increased production of interleukin-6, an immune-system messenger. This coincides with research findings indicating that stress and depression have a negative effect on the immune system. Reduced immunity makes the body more susceptible to everything from colds and flus to cancer. For example, the incidence of serious illness, including cancer, is significantly higher among people who have suffered the death of a spouse in the previous year. Fortunately, this immune-suppression process can be corrected with psychotherapy, medication, or any number of other positive influences that restore hope and a feeling of self-esteem. The ability of human beings to recover from adversity is remarkable.

# Anxiety

Though the general population may often use the terms stress and anxiety interchangeably, it may be helpful to make some distinctions. While stress may refer to both stimulus and response, anxiety describes only our response, often when the stimulus is not even present. Though it may not be pleasant, anxiety is not necessarily bad. The feeling of apprehension—the gnawing feeling in the pit of the stomach that "something is wrong"—is a natural warning signal. Appropriate concern leads us to study and to pay our bills on time. When appropriate, anxiety, like good stress ("eustress" according to Selye), is a coordinated group of reactions that prepare a person to respond to a perceived threat.

Anxiety, however, usually refers to the thoughts, feelings, physical sensations, and behaviors associated with worry and fear. According to psychologist Judy Eidelson and psychiatrist David Burns, ". . . depression is the certainty that things are horrible and hopeless; anxiety is the belief that at any moment things will become horrible and hopeless."[8]

Anxious thoughts range from realistic concern to inappropriate preoccupations. The primary emotion in anxiety is clearly fear, though it can include others, from anticipatory excitement to depression. The simplest physical sensation is an inner uneasiness, which can grow to be severe. Anxious feelings may intensify when we worry about a specific event, and may include physical sensations such as dry mouth, sweaty palms, or queasy stomach. Behaviorally, anxiety often triggers exaggerated motor activity, from increased breathing rate and restlessness to pacing and insomnia.

## Anxiety Disorder

One in 10 Americans will experience an anxiety disorder that will cause impairment in functioning at some point in their lives. When anxiety habitually persists or intensifies out of proportion to situations, it is labeled an "anxiety disorder." An episode of anxiety severe enough to interfere with a person's ability to function is referred to as a "panic attack," and is often accompanied by palpitations, chest pain, feelings of light-headedness, and fear of death. Five percent of women and 2% of men will experience anxiety disorder at some point in their lives.

## Phobias

An intense and unreasonable fear of certain objects or situations is called a *phobia*. People can have phobias of anything in life—from insects and height, to sex or flying. Some pathologically anxious individuals stay at home rather than risk exposure to any situation out of their control. The fear that leads them to avoid open areas or crowds is called *agoraphobia*, literally "fear of the marketplace." Seven percent of women will experience agoraphobia at some point in their lives; twice as many as men. Social phobia is a persistent fear of social situations in which one might become embarrassed. According to the Diagnostic and Statistical Manual-IV (DSM-IV) of the psychiatric and medical professions, anywhere from 3% to 20% of the population has some degree of social phobia, depending on the threshold used to determine distress.[9] Fifteen percent of women will experience social phobia at some point in their lives. For men, the rate is 11%.[10]

## Chronic Anxiety

With continued stress, anxiety can become chronic and habitual, and can actually impair one's ability to handle the stress. Some people suffer from "free-floating anxiety," a profoundly uncomfortable sense of acute worry, which the person is unable to relate to a specific cause. Besides being a destabilizing influence in and of itself, this condition also predisposes the individual to respond poorly to stressful situations in general.

### Obsessive-Compulsive Disorder

Someone with "Obsessive-Compulsive Disorder" (OCD) suffers extreme anxiety and stress brought on by recurring intrusive and inappropriate thoughts or images, and compulsive and repetitive behaviors. Common examples of such thoughts are fears of contamination, fear of making harmful mistakes, or fear of a partner's unfaithfulness. Compulsive behaviors seem driven by unreasonable fears, and might appear to be acting out extreme superstitions. Jack Nicholson's Academy Award®-winning role in *As Good As It Gets* displayed many of the characteristic behaviors of OCD—excessive hand washing, repetitive turning of doorknobs and locks, and rituals of avoiding the lines in the sidewalk. Most people with OCD fully recognize that their thoughts and behaviors are inappropriate, but feel powerless to stop them. OCD affects about 6 million people annually—as many as asthma or diabetes.

## Our External and Internal Stressors

Even without a crisis, the body undergoes periods of physical stress. Some of these are of our own making, caused by smoking, excessive eating, consistent late nights, or lack of exercise. External stressors can be as varied as loud noise, secondhand smoke, atmospheric pollution, chemical food additives, or poor nutrition. As we go through life, most of us learn to adapt successfully to these stimuli. Nevertheless they take their toll.

Contemporary society is marked by four widespread sources of anxiety. Due to actual and perceived increases in crime and violence, we are more afraid. Due to rapidly shifting and uncertain job markets, we are insecure. In all areas

## The Various Symptoms of Anxiety

Physical symptoms of anxiety

| | |
|---|---|
| Recurring headaches | Vague aches and pains |
| Dizziness | Heartburn |
| Muscle tension | Ringing in the ears |
| Dry mouth | Flushing |
| Excessive perspiration | Pounding heart |
| Insomnia | Palpitations |
| Fatigue | |

Psychological and behavioral symptoms of anxiety

| | |
|---|---|
| Irritability | Loss of libido |
| Loss of concentration | Excessive smoking |
| Restlessness | Alcohol craving/ |
| Loss of memory | excessive drinking |
| Lack of motivation | |

Emotional symptoms of anxiety

| | |
|---|---|
| Worry | Increased guilt or shame |
| Nervousness | Fear of doom and dying |
| Exaggerated self-awareness | Panic[11] |

of our lives, we constantly confront pervasive and accelerating change. Finally, supportive relationships are probably the single best protector against the ravages of stress, yet due to mobility and the breakdown of family and community, we have never been more alone.

We are socially conditioned, almost from birth, to react to stress in a way that exacerbates rather than relieves it. In a more rational, reasonable world, we would be lovingly guided and nurtured to help overcome our predisposition toward the stress response. Instead, we are encouraged to deny fear and hold back anger, which only worsens the hand nature has dealt us. Stress disempowers and limits us, narrowing our view of what's possible in our jobs, our relationships, and our society.

## It's Not the Stimulus, It's the Response

Is there any way out of this disabling pattern? Scientific research—and our own experience (if we only take the time to notice)—reveal that the answer lies not in our environment, but within ourselves. "How is this possible?" you might ask. "The stress is real, it's everywhere. It's beyond my control!"

Or is it? The mind is a miraculous phenomenon. Truth is as we perceive it. Imagine how many times a day you are certain that you have seen or experienced an event one way, when someone else (or even you in another frame of mind) experiences it quite differently. For example, in a cranky mood, while dining at a restaurant, you could feel annoyed at hearing raucous laughter coming from the next table. In a more gregarious mood, you would happily engage in some playful banter with those same noisy neighbors.

- The bad news is: We create our own stress
- The good news is: We create our own stress

It is not the event itself that hurts us, but how we interpret it. How we respond to the events of life determines whether we become victims or winners as a result of the stressors in our modern jungle. We will talk more about this in later chapters.

# Toward a Holistic Perspective

In the next chapter, we will examine the physiological aspects of stress and anxiety, and their enormous implications for our physical health. We will also explore the concept of the mind–body continuum, looking in the "opposite direction" for the medical causes of anxiety and depression.

## CHAPTER 3

# Stress and Disease: The Mind–Body Continuum

Western medicine, and Western thought in general, has presumed a division between mind and body. The divisions are not so clear-cut, however, and the body and mind actually work as an integrated whole. This means that any trauma or stress, whether mental or physical, will affect all systems. This chapter addresses the enormous impact of stress on our physical health, and then looks at this relationship from the other side, examining the effects of medical problems and metabolic imbalances on our mental health.

## Anxiety and Brain Chemistry

Regardless of the triggering factors, the underlying mechanism of anxiety or depression is a shift in brain chemistry. The brain is made up of nerve cells or *neurons*. Between the neurons are small gaps called *synapses.* In order for a message to pass from one neuron to its neighbor across the synapse, a chemical messenger called a *neurotransmitter* is released. The pre-synaptic neuron—the one that is sending the message—produces the neurotransmitter, which moves toward the post-synaptic neuron on the receiving end. The neurotransmitter molecule can be pictured as a key that will fit only a certain lock—called its receptor site—on the post-synaptic neuron. When the matching key slides into the lock, the message has been received, and the receptor is either activated or inhibited, depending on its function.

Once its job is complete, the neurotransmitter molecule is released back into the synapse. It might return to the precursor neuron where it can be used again. Or, it might remain in the synapse along with other chemical messengers. The molecule may then continue the cycle by reconnecting with another receptor, or it may be inactivated by an enzyme, one of which is *monoamine oxidase* (MAO).

Our moods are affected by changes in the relative levels of various neurotransmitters. Shifts in the sensitivity level of the receptor site in relation to the neurotransmitter also play a role. The interaction of neurotransmitters and mood works both ways as well. Chemical influences or medications aside, we can actually alter the balance of our neurotransmitters with a change in mood.

## Serotonin and Other
## Mood-Affecting Substances

---

*Serotonin* is one of the major neurotransmitters, influencing many physiological functions, including blood pressure, digestion, body temperature, and pain sensation. It also affects circadian rhythm (the body's response to the cycles of day and night) as well as mood. Low levels of serotonin are associated with:

- Depression
- Obsessive thinking
- Anxiety
- Increased sensitivity to pain
- Emotional volatility, including violent behavior against self and others
- Alcohol and drug abuse
- Premenstrual syndrome (PMS)
- Increased sexual desire
- Carbohydrate cravings
- Sleep disturbances

On the other hand, healthy levels of serotonin are associated with emotional and social stability. The antidepressant effects of the Prozac-like drugs and, most likely, the herb St. John's wort, are due to their ability to raise serotonin levels.

## Endorphins: Our Internal Tranquilizers

The brain produces hormones called *endorphins* to keep us tranquil and pain-free in the face of life's uncertainties. Endorphins are similar in structure to morphine and heroin, functioning like natural opiates in our brains and producing pleasurable feelings such as a "runner's high." Receptors in the brain receive these hormones and respond to their signals. Again, like locks and keys, when the right hormone is present, the receptor shuts off its signals, producing tranquility or pain relief.

Stress can increase anxiety through two mechanisms that upset the brain's balance of these "natural tranquilizers." As stress levels rise and become protracted, the brain increases its production of these hormones to protect us during an emergency. If the stress continues, however, the brain begins to shut down the supply. There is a natural protective system at work. Both pain and anxiety increase as stress persists, as a way of telling us to quit doing that which damages us. If our bodies didn't do this, the more stress we created, the more peaceful we would feel, and that would probably interfere with our chances of survival.

The second mechanism that can increase anxiety involves the stress hormone cortisol, which is produced by the adrenal glands in almost direct proportion to adrenaline (see Chapter 2). When we're under stress, however, cortisol production in the brain increases to such an extent that it forms a barrier to the brain's natural tranquilizers, blocking them from reaching their receptors. Inability to access endorphins as a response to prolonged stress can result in high anxiety and eventually panic attacks, or even a downward spiral into depression. In addition, prolonged exposure to cortisol can actually destroy brain cells.

If anxiety can be costly and dangerous, why isn't the regulatory mechanism adjusted so that it is expressed only when danger is actually present? Unfortunately, in many situations it is not clear whether or not anxiety is needed. Our bodies mobilize for danger far too often because even once, the cost of getting killed seems enormously higher than the cost of responding to a hundred false alarms.

This was demonstrated by an experiment in which guppies were separated into timid, ordinary, and bold groups on the basis of their reactions when confronted by a small-mouth bass: hiding, swimming away, or eyeing the intruder. Each group of guppies was then left in a tank with a bass. After sixty hours, 40% of the timid guppies and 15% of the ordinary guppies were still there, but *none of the bold guppies had survived.*[1] Perhaps the bold guppies could have used a little more anxiety.

## The Effects of Stress on Our Health

Since our bodies are designed to react to intermittent physical stress rather than constant mental or emotional stress, prolonged stress, with no relief in sight, places an enormous burden on all systems. Disease is the inevitable outcome.

According to the American Heart Association, more than 25% of Americans suffer from essential hypertension (high blood pressure). One out of every two deaths in the United States is caused by some form of heart or vascular disease. In the 1980s, researchers at the National Institutes of Health found that an important precursor to developing heart disease was "emotional toxicity"—or how we react emotionally to the events in our lives. Men who are incapable of relaxing after work have a risk of heart attack nearly three times greater than those who say they can relax and forget about their work. Those who are able to create a strong sense of belonging and connection with others have fewer diseases and less stress. Those who have altruistic beliefs and behavior are more resistant to stress and chronic disease.[2]

## The Mind–Body Continuum:
## It Works Both Ways

As we have seen, mental and emotional stress can have enormous repercussions on our physical health. Once we understand such interactions within the mind-body, it only makes sense that the reverse is true as well. While psychological symptoms can signify an unresolved emotional issue, they

## Table 3.1   The Effects of Stress on Systems in the Body

Central Nervous System
- Anxiety, depression, and fatigue

Cardiovascular System
- Impaired heart function; can cause angina
- Constriction of the peripheral blood vessels, thereby raising blood pressure

Digestive System
- Stomach upsets, even ulcers
- Diarrhea
- Gastritis
- Peptic ulcers
- Irritable Bowel Syndrome
- Colitis
- Canker sores in the mouth

Respiratory System
- Asthma

Musculoskeletal System
- Tension in skeletal muscles and joints, leading to backache and muscular aches and pains
- Predisposition to arthritis; degenerative diseases such as rheumatoid arthritis

can also be the result of a brain chemistry imbalance, including one caused by a diagnosable medical illness. We can approach the biochemical causes of anxiety from two vantage points. One involves physical disorders and their effects on mental health, and the other involves the chemistry of the brain itself.

Good health depends on both a healthy body and a healthy mind. Therefore, it is senseless to expect the brain to work correctly without the rest of the body being in proper balance. Every disorder or deficiency in the body

Immune System
- Weakened defenses, with lowered resistance to infections
- Viral illnesses (often due to a depleted immune defense system)
- Allergies
- Malignant cell changes; cancer

Endocrine System
- Menstrual disorders
- Thyroid disorders (underactive, overactive, thyroiditis)
- Adrenal hypofunction

Reproductive System
- Infertility
- Premature ejaculation
- Impotence

Skin
- Eczema, psoriasis, rashes

General
- Tissue degeneration
- Acceleration of aging process

affects the brain, which is extremely sensitive to metabolic imbalances caused by such physical problems as low blood sugar, water retention, or oxygen deprivation. Often, people who are not responding to psychotherapy show accelerated improvement once their metabolic conditions are properly diagnosed and treated.

Conventional medicine often fails to look at these factors. If the doctor is unaware of the deeper connection between body chemistry and illness, he or she will never test for these elements, and an opportunity for healing will be

## Body Knowledge Resolves "Mind" Illnesses

The importance of the mind-body connection has not always been recognized, sometimes resulting in tragic consequences. Take, for example a disorder called *cretinism*, which is rare today. Severely retarded from birth, children born with cretinism were doomed to lives of miserable dependency, often in crowded institutions. Finally, it was discovered that they were deficient in thyroid hormone due to a lack of iodine intake by their mothers during pregnancy. Without this needed mineral during gestation, their thyroid glands could not develop normally, resulting in retardation. The solution was iodized salt, which is now a legislated dietary supplement. Rather than a genetic, irreversible illness, cretinism was simply an unrecognized mineral deficiency that could be treated once the dietary link was discovered.

Another example of a physical illness masquerading as a mental illness is *pellagra*. During the nineteenth and early twentieth centuries, mental institutions were filled with demented pellagra patients. Researchers eventually discovered that this severe mental illness could be reversed—or prevented—through the administration of vitamin $B_3$ (Niacin). Although pellagra is a physical disease, the first

lost. Holistically oriented physicians, however, look further, aware that anxiety can be a signal of a malfunction in the mind-body continuum as we saw in Table 3.1 on page 34.

An acknowledged innovator in alternative medicine, endocrinologist and author Deepak Chopra writes, ". . . mind and body are like parallel universes, and the latest discoveries in neurobiology build an even stronger case. . . . Anything and most prominent symptoms are mental in nature. Once doctors recognized the true origin of the disease, pellagra patients all but disappeared from mental hospitals.

A continuation of this science of treating illnesses as an imbalance in body chemistry is found in the practice of "orthomolecular medicine." A term coined by Nobel Prize-winning researcher Linus Pauling, *orthomolecular* means the right molecule in the right place. The medical profession continues to make these important discoveries. In the 1950s, pioneers in the field of orthomolecular psychiatry, Dr. Abram Hoffer and Dr. Humphrey Osmond, noticed that many people with schizophrenia responded well to high doses of niacin. The psychiatric establishment, however, would not accept these remarkable findings, and soon the advent of the major tranquilizers left this discovery behind. While the pharmaceutical industry profited from these drugs, the root cause and simple solution to some schizophrenia cases were ignored. It is still a viable treatment for those fortunate enough to get help from orthomolecular physicians. There are many conditions like this, some certainly yet to be discovered.

that happens in the mental universe must leave tracks in the physical one."[3] In other words, human beings live as "open systems." Open systems are characterized by options and creative expression. We constantly interact with our environment, change it, and in turn are changed by it. We have the capacity to create chaos or harmony, to be self-destructive, or to create wellness and fulfillment. We can

**Table 3.2    Medical Causes of Anxiety**

Metabolic Disorders
* These include hypoglycemia (low blood sugar), premenstrual syndrome (PMS), and food and chemical sensitivities.

Nutritional Deficiencies
* These include lack of vitamins, minerals, or amino acids, caused by poor diet, malabsorption, or anorexia.

Hormonal Imbalances
* These include problems in the pituitary, pineal, thyroid, or adrenal glands; imbalances in sex hormones; or any combination of these.

Toxins
* These include substances of abuse, especially withdrawal from stimulants such as caffeine, nicotine, cocaine, or depressants such as alcohol or heroin; heavy metals, including lead and mercury; and chemicals, including petroleum products such as PCBs (used in making plastics, solvents, and pesticides).

Side Effects of Prescribed Medication (partial list)
* This includes antidepressants such as Prozac; incorrect doses of thyroid medication; and habituation and withdrawal effects related to the benzodiazepines, antianxiety drugs, which are discussed in Chapter 5.

choose to eat properly, drive carefully, balance our work with our leisure, and take control of our emotional lives.

# Research on the Mind–Body Connection

Researchers find that daily small pleasurable events, such as a pleasant family celebration or having friends over, strengthen the immune system for the next one or two days. On the other hand, unpleasant daily experiences, such as work pressures or an argument with your spouse, weaken the immune system on the day of the event.[4]

# Medical Sources of Anxiety and Depression

Medical illness causes anxiety and depression more often than many doctors think. It should be routinely suspected before assuming the symptoms are simply psychological. Anxiety is often an initial symptom of disorders such as hyperthyroidism, heart disease, anemia, and adrenal tumors, as we saw in Table 3.2 on page 38. Since the mind and body together form a complex interactive system, several of these biological factors may occur at once. Imbalance in one area often leads to imbalance in another, requiring a careful sifting through the various signs and symptoms to arrive at a correct diagnosis and treatment. (Nutritional supplementation will be covered in greater detail in Chapter 13.)

# Below the Surface

In the next two chapters, we will look at the two primary conventional treatments for the complex problems of stress and anxiety: Psychotherapy and pharmaceutical drugs. The next chapter examines some of the underlying sources of these problems and introduces some therapeutic techniques I have found particularly effective.

## CHAPTER 4

# Anxiety: Psychological Factors

The way each of us handles stress, and the level of anxiety that results, is determined by multiple factors. We begin with our genetic endowment; our inborn tendencies. Added to that are the psychological, physical, and biochemical influences of our environment. All these factors play a role in how we ultimately feel and respond.

## Genetic

We all start with our genetic background: the built-in blueprint of "who we are to be." Aside from any environmental influences, certain genetic factors predispose individuals to anxiety. The tendency for panic disorder, for example, runs in families.[1] This does not mean that having an anxiety disorder is inevitable. Rather, it is one of many factors that affect your ability to respond to anxiety-producing events. In twin studies, which give a good indication of the effect of nature vs. nurture, panic attacks were concordant in 31% of identical twins, and 0% in fraternal twins. That is, in 69% of the cases, only one twin had panic attacks, despite identical genetic make-up.[2] As in the case of identical twins who did not have the disorder, we can do much to help ourselves in this area, as discussed in this chapter.

# Psychological Factors:
# The Effects of Trauma

What roles do environment, early experiences, and trauma play in the development of anxiety? Research has clearly shown that not only will certain stressors cause anxiety as a direct response, but repeated stress may predispose an individual to future episodes of both anxiety and depression. In addition to any genetic predisposition, actual chemical changes occur in the brain in response to trauma, making the person more vulnerable to such events in the future.

Trauma need not be physical or obvious. While there may be no overt physical abuse, there may be ongoing psychological abuse, from overt bullying to subtle shaming, criticism, and lack of emotional support. Many children experience such abuse on numerous levels every day of their lives from those that they trust the most—their parents, other family members, teachers, and other authority figures. Raised by well-meaning but misguided parents, they may carry old messages of "life as performance" and "not measuring up." The inner need to be perfect, to be pleasing, to not express one's true feelings can hang over us throughout our lives. A lack of love and support during childhood can cause emotional scarring that, if left untreated, lasts into and throughout adulthood.

According to researcher Peter Levine in his book *Waking the Tiger Within,* any type of abuse, whether physical or emotional, can produce effects on the psyche and brain chemistry, leading to chronic anxiety and depression.[3] The fear engendered by this continuum of experiences does not disappear. It lives within us, affecting our minds, emotions, and behavior as if it were happening today. Our entire culture—from school systems, to advertising, to the workplace—is built around these fears. This environment creates more stress, with constant inner comparisons, negative self-talk, and a perpetual inner anxiety. Thus, even if your present-day problems seem under control, old ones will continue to pop up in other guises as long as the inner patterns remain unresolved. The target of these worries in the body is the inner seat of fear and anxiety: the adrenal glands (see Chapter 3 on how the adrenal glands affect our brain and body chemistry).

## Post-Traumatic Stress Disorder

Throughout our lives, negative experiences can produce still further damage. You may be familiar with the problems of certain war veterans, or victims of assault, who suffer from post-traumatic stress disorder (PTSD). This condition stems from an event that threatens death or serious injury to the individual or others. Its sufferers are generally depressed, anxious, and irritable. They have difficulty concentrating, suffer from sleep disturbances, have an exaggerated "startle response," experience a variety of physical complaints, and have difficulty maintaining jobs and relationships. They often suffer from attacks of unreasonable rage and violence that are out of proportion with any current provocation.

How does this happen? Violence, threat of violence, or a similar experience make an indelible mark on the psyche. As we discussed earlier, actual chemical changes occur in the brain that correspond to these psychological traumas. The ability to maintain emotional balance is destroyed. PTSD sufferers' lives become increasingly difficult, even impossible, for both them and their loved ones. These individuals experience a high rate of family and marital problems, divorce, chronic illness, and suicide. Similar syndromes are seen in survivors of other traumas, such as people who have lost their homes in fires, or victims of assault or rape.

While these cases are extreme and the cause is apparent, many other people are similarly affected by early cumulative abuse, and live in a state of heightened anxiety, tension, depression, and despair. This includes people who appear to have "free-floating anxiety" with no apparent cause. They are often treated with medication, which never gives them a chance to heal these old wounds. This is like treating a bursting appendix with painkillers. You might dull the pain, but the patient needs immediate surgery to save his or her life. The pain is a signal of a serious problem, and masking the pain could be fatal. Likewise, treating all emotional problems with prescription medication is not the answer. While it may relieve some immediate pain, the underlying problem will continue to fester under the surface, like an inflamed appendix, until the individual gets to the root of the problem. Following is a good example of this situation from my own practice.

## A Case of Trauma, EMDR, and Benzo Withdrawal

### *Background*

Don, a 45-year-old convenience-store manager, came to see me, saying he was "disgusted with the pill-pushing psychiatrists at the clinic" (referring to his HMO's mental health center). Don told me, "I'm hooked on these drugs. I want to get off them and try something more natural." I sympathized with him, while also understanding doctors' overloaded schedules and impossibly large doctor-patient ratios which left them no time to administer much-needed psychotherapy. Their only tools seem to be prescription medications. Don had been given alprazolam (Xanax) daily for anxiety; temazepam (Restoril) every night for sleep; and an antidepressant, Trazodone. "I used to get mean and cranky at times, but now I don't even have the energy for that. I'm so depressed, life doesn't seem worth living. But I'm a religious man and can't even consider suicide. And I love my wife. That would kill her," Don said. His problems were compounded by the loss of sexual desire he had experienced ever since he began taking the medications three years earlier.

## Treatment

The drugs were no longer effective, but Don was strongly addicted to them. Discontinuing them too rapidly could be dangerous, and withdrawal must be undertaken under medical supervision. I placed Don on a very gradually decreasing dose of his medications, while adding a supplement program for anxiety that included kava, the amino acids GABA and glutamine, and the herb valerian, all of which have calming effects. I added St. John's wort as well, an excellent herb for anxiety, depression, and insomnia (see Chapter 12). St. John's wort can take anywhere from one to six weeks to become fully effective. The other supplements would begin to work immediately, dealing with any signs of withdrawal, and helping him to transition off the medication and on to nonaddictive, natural substances.

I learned that three years earlier, Don had been the victim of an armed robbery at his store, during which a coworker had been shot to death. Despite the years that had passed since then, it was clear that Don was in great need of psychotherapy to deal with his trauma. In our minds, time is always in the present tense, and past hurts can affect us as much today as when they first occurred. We began by using Eye Movement Desensitization and Reprocessing (EMDR), developed by psychologist Francine Shapiro.[4] With this technique, an individual recalls and reexperiences an earlier traumatic incident in a safe setting, allowing the mind to fully experience and release suppressed emotions.

In the course of our work together, I asked Don to picture the robbery scene. He recalled the terror, the thoughts of his wife and children whom he might never see again, and the utter helplessness of his situation. As he focused on his feelings, I asked him to follow my fingers with his eyes in a rapid back-and-forth motion. He soon was in tears, recalling further details of the event. We persisted with the eye movements. He went through an entire movie in his head: seeing the hold-up; handing over the money; being bound, gagged, and left on the floor; and witnessing his employee being fatally shot. His overriding feeling was, "I'm helpless. It's my fault," as if he could have prevented the incident or saved his friend. He felt guilty and ashamed.

As we continued, I asked Don to consider a different perspective on the event, and his responsibility for it. He soon realized that he had done his best, and that he was, in fact, lucky to have survived. Our work together allowed him to fully experience, process, and let go of these tormenting feelings. His body relaxed, he began to laugh through his tears, and exclaimed, "Of course it wasn't my fault! I did the best I could. I do deserve to live!"

In subsequent visits, he revealed that he had been mistreated as a child by his army officer father, for whom he could "never do it quite right." He felt that no matter how hard he tried, he wasn't the "perfect little man" that he was expected to be. This abusive underpinning to his future ordeal had slanted his perspective, which our work together helped to rectify. In the process of dealing with an adult trauma, he was able to access and heal his childhood wounds. This bonus is common in therapy. Once the roots of the current problem are discovered and healed, the person becomes better or more whole than they had ever been *before* the adult trauma.

———————————

How does trauma affect someone so profoundly, and for so long? The most likely explanation is as follows: The early abuse put Don's emotional memory bank, like an inner recorder or VCR, on pause. EMDR, which induces rapid eye movements, allowed his VCR to release and move through the old film and into the present. The rapid eye movement of EMDR is similar to what occurs during dream sleep. Emotional leftovers of the day are processed neatly by our brains through our dreams, and EMDR seems to be a way of producing the same healing function. Preliminary research indicates that psychotherapy actually produces corresponding changes in brain chemistry. The early experiences likely affected his brain chemistry, leaving him more vulnerable to future trauma. Moreover, the medication he had been taking suppressed REM sleep, not allowing him the depth of sleep and the time periods of processing and integration that everyone needs each night to maintain emotional equilibrium.

As in Don's case, symptoms may be evidence of buried emotional wounds that can haunt an individual until they are uncovered and processed. The idea of treating symptoms alone, without looking underneath for the root cause, is shortsighted and ultimately, ineffective. During my years of practice, I have found that the best way to help patients deal with a difficult feeling is to encourage them to go right into it, embrace it, and see what is behind it. Much of the emotional pain we experience may actually be a result of our attempts to resist it! We may reflexively try to shut it out, which only forces it underground, haunting us in disguise as depression, anxiety, headaches, or even serious illness.

The solution? Instead of seeing painful feelings— or illnesses—as enemies, see them as messages from the unconscious mind and even the body. Ignoring or turning off such signals can be a dangerous thing, like unplugging a smoke alarm when it starts to beep. Common sense tells us we should instead look for the fire that's the source of the smoke. The use of medication such as the benzodiazepines are particularly problematic here, because they do not do a good job of handling the anxiety. They certainly can't treat the source, and often lead to further anxiety and depression as well as other unwanted side effects. In many cases, the patient becomes addicted to the drug.

Don's treatment of a long-term, gradual withdrawal from medication and a regimen of nutritional supplements went extremely well. Because of the therapy, and his dealing definitively with the source of his anxiety, we were able to address the medication issue largely from a physiological angle. He felt stronger psychologically, was eager to become independent of the drugs, and had the inner tools to deal with any anxiety that did crop up. Over a few months time, he was able to stop all medication, while remaining on a natural supplement program.

Don was proud of himself and felt like a "real man" perhaps for the first time. We were not simply substituting herbs and amino acids for drugs. Rather, the herbal supplements were helping to correct an imbalance in his brain chemistry that resulted from both his early trauma and his medication use. Unlike his experience with the medication, while taking the herbs, he was still able to have a full range of normal emotions—from joy to sadness, even some "normal" anxiety at times. The difference was that he was no longer a victim of either his emotions, the chemical imbalance perpetuated by the drugs, or his addiction to them. And by the way, he was also able to return to a healthy sex life.

A preliminary study on the use of kava as a bridge in benzodiazepine withdrawal is being conducted. While no results are yet available, the project is promising. I have had good results in using it, as illustrated by Don's story.

## The Inner Voices of Stress

A useful way of looking at the psychology of stress is to examine the various subpersonalities that live in our minds. Do I mean that we are all multiple personalities? Sometimes it sure seems like it! Have you ever had an internal dialogue such as the one in the following paragraphs?

It's a workday, and you have stepped out of bed and peered outside to check the weather, which happens to be beautiful. You think to yourself, "I'd sure enjoy going to the beach today. The sun's shining, there's a warm breeze, and I would love to work on my tan!" You consider calling in sick. After all, the office has been slow lately, and you could always make up the work later. Then, your inner voice of responsibility comes slamming down on your growing fantasy: "No way. You are due at the office in an hour, and there's no way you're not going to show up!"

You dutifully drop the alternate plan, and get ready for work, wistfully considering the possibilities for the weekend. Your "Inner Player" didn't have a chance against the "Inner Good Girl"—the voice of duty and responsibility. Social conditioning rightly takes the form of inner voices like hers. Without those inner voices, we would act on every childlike impulse. On the other hand, our Inner Player needs space too. What we need is a balance, decided upon by a mature "Inner Self" who weighs the options, considers the pros and cons, and takes action. We develop these inner voices or subpersonalities early in life, based on the dictates of our parents, teachers, and other societal influences. When there is conflict among the voices, we experience inner stress, confusion, and even chaos.

## Karin's Voices

### Background

My patient, Karin, was well aware of her own dynamics. A successful film producer, she was between projects. However, she complained that despite not having to be anywhere or do anything in particular—an enviable position for anyone—she felt restless, anxious, and as if she ought to be "doing something." Even sitting down to read a book in the middle of the day made her feel guilty.

## Treatment

I used a technique called Voice Dialogue, which consists of the therapist actually addressing these voices or subpersonalities and offering them an empathetic ear. I checked in with her "Inner Pusher" (her inner controller or boss) who was being fed by her "Inner Critic." The "Pusher/Critic" said, "She's lazy, so I have to be the enforcer. She'd like to hang out and play. But she's here for a purpose. She thinks life is supposed to be fun, but she needs to be prepared for life's problems. I'm the one who helps her keep up with information and issues, and helps run her life. Otherwise, she'd be a bum, just like her father [who had left the family when Karin was six]. He had a good time, and look what happened to him." Karin's role model was always her hardworking mother.

Karin's response to this inner voice was, "The 'Pusher' doesn't think I'll survive without him. It's like a war zone, it's so intense. He doesn't trust me, and he's always warning me about something." (Our inner voices can be male or female—which ever they seem to us.) "I guess he did get me through boot camp [referring to her difficult childhood]. I'm OK now, though. I survived."

I asked the "Pusher/Critic" what motivated him. He responded, "I only meant to help her. It was never my intention for her to have a stressful life. She never told me she didn't need me. We've been going by the old script. I never knew people could learn and choose. This is eye-opening. I'm glad to be able to come out and be heard. What should I do now?" He continued, "She feels obligated to me, since I've been so helpful in the past. But she can take my advice or leave it—it won't hurt my feelings."

## Results

A month later, I checked in with Karin's "Inner Child," asking how *she* was feeling. The "Inner Child" told me, "Life has been pretty good lately. Even though Karin is working hard on a new project, she makes time to go for walks with me.

Sometimes when she's working, she talks to me. She used to just ignore me. She's a lot less stressed now than she was before. Sometimes, though, she forgets about me, and I get sad. She feels it, too, and knows that I need some attention. We're reading stories again, a chapter at a time. I love books."

Karin, the whole person, and not one of these parts or voices, commented, "It's so nice to talk to these personalities. It's much easier when I understand what's going on. When I want to read, which my "Child" loves, my "Pusher" wants me to work in order to survive and be successful. Well, I *am* successful, and I can choose my activities. I can be in control of myself by *listening* to these voices, instead of either blindly obeying or ignoring them! When the "Pusher" comes on really strong, I take a little kava. My "Inner Child" says it makes it easier for her to get my attention."

---

Karin became more aware of her inner dialogue through my participation as facilitator. However, this inner conversation goes on in all of us all the time. The awareness of these different parts with different scripts or needs can help us to resolve tension. Simply acknowledging the conflict by listening to each of the voices can be healing. If we can't communicate with ourselves, how can we ever hope to communicate with others? We see here how perception is relative. Which of our "selves" is observing? Which one is experiencing? Who should have the last word? How do we compromise? Just as in Karin's case, it is up to us to use the voices as we wish, instead of accepting their conflicting demands at face value.

We see from Karin's story that if we ignore the "Inner Child," we are setting ourselves up for stress. Instead, we can allow our "Inner Child" to be the stress meter, letting us know when it's time to relax. In this way, we can keep from losing our spontaneity, our playfulness, and ultimately, our health. Stress can arise from the actions of the "Inner Critic"—that voice for whom we are never good enough—which causes us to feel worthless or guilty, despite our accomplishments.

Often, successful type-A people don't know what to do with themselves on vacation. Work, though stressful, is their drug of choice. Their task, like Karin's, is to put the "Pusher" aside at times, and connect with their "Child."

Voice Dialogue therapy, as demonstrated here, was developed by Drs. Hal Stone and Sidra Stone, who have written several books on the subject.[5] It has been an important tool in my practice and in my own life for many years.

In the next chapter we will look at the role of medications in treating stress and anxiety, why they are prescribed so readily, and the enormous drawbacks of their use and abuse: Side-effects, tolerance, and addiction. Finally, we will introduce the possibility of natural alternatives, particularly kava.

## CHAPTER 5

# Medications:
# The Antidepressants
# and Tranquilizers

**D**ebra, a 27-year-old store clerk, sat across from mc, sounding hopeless, and told me the following story. She had been suffering from anxiety and depression, which had worsened over the past year, and finally led her to consult a psychiatrist. "First, the doctor put me on Paxil for my nerves, which zonked me out—I was walking around like a zombie. So he switched me to Zoloft. It was okay for the first few weeks, but then I realized that my sex life had disappeared—I just wasn't interested any more. My husband was not pleased, either. Then I noticed that I was more nervous than ever, and had trouble sleeping. When the doctor suggested I take two different tranquilizers (Klonopin for the anxiety and Restoril for sleep), I just gave up. I was not going to spend the rest of my life on pills! I threw them all away and decided there had to be a better way."

There *was* a better way, as you will see in the following chapters. As shown in Debra's case, the common medical treatments for anxiety and insomnia are prescriptions for antidepressants, such as Paxil and Zoloft, and for antianxiety agents, the most common being the benzodiazepines, such as Xanax, Klonopin, and Restoril.

# Antidepressants

Beginning in the 1950s, scientists developed a number of synthetic drugs for the treatment of depression, which represented a major step forward at the time. In the 1980s, the selective serotonin re-uptake inhibitors (SSRIs) arrived on the scene, with substantially different, perhaps more tolerable, side effects than the older tricyclics. There are now three principal types of antidepressant medications: the tricyclic drugs, the monoamine oxidase inhibitors (MAOIs), and the selective serotonin re-uptake inhibitors (SSRIs). There are also three drugs that are chemically distinct from these types and each other: Wellbutrin, Desyrel, and Effexor. The drugs differ in their mechanisms of action and side effects; however, they all have several things in common. They are effective in reducing anxiety and depressive symptoms in 60% to 80% of the persons who use them. They also take from a month to six weeks to produce their full effects, although changes in mood can occur much sooner. And they all have side effects, some of which are serious.

## The Tricyclics

The first antidepressant medications, which are still used today, are the tricyclics. They include imipramine hydrochloride (Tofranil), clomipramine (Anafranil), amitriptyline hydrochloride (Elavil, Limbitrol, Endep), desipramine hydrochloride (Norpramin), doxepin hydrochloride (Adapin, Sinequan), nortriptyline hydrochloride (Pamelor, Aventyl), and protriptyline hydrochloride (Vivactil). The tricyclics work by increasing the level of neurotransmitters—the chemical messengers in the brain that elevate mood. A serious problem with the tricyclics is their side effects, which include blood pressure changes, drowsiness, arrhythmias (irregularities in heartbeat), sedation, dry mouth, blurred vision, confusion, weight gain, flulike symptoms, sweating, rashes, nausea, constipation or diarrhea, difficulty with urination, impotence or impaired erection in men, inhibited orgasm in women, nightmares, and anxiety.

Due to these effects, tricyclics are not usually prescribed, except when the sedation they cause is desirable. Cost is also a consideration, since they are considerably cheaper than the SSRIs. Some doctors will prescribe either doxepin or desipramine to be taken at bedtime for their sedative effect in order to counter the insomnia that often occurs with Prozac. Anafranil is often prescribed for obsessive-compulsive disorder, or the SSRIs Prozac, Luvox, or Zoloft may be prescribed, if the side effects of the tricyclics are a problem.

### The Monoamine Oxidase Inhibitors

The monoamine oxidase inhibitors (MAOs), which include phenelzine sulfate (Nardil) and tranylcypromine sulfate (Parnate), are seldom used today because they are dangerous. They work by inhibiting the enzyme MAO within the synapse, leading to a greater supply of neurotransmitters in the synapse, and resulting in a reduction of depressive symptoms. Some common side effects include insomnia, impotence and other sexual dysfunction, dizziness, weight gain, and water retention. They can also produce a dangerous elevation in blood pressure, if the patient consumes substances containing the amino acid tyramine, such as aged wine or cheese, or many of the common cold remedies.

### The Selective Serotonin Re-Uptake Inhibitors

Prozac (fluoxetine hydrochloride) was the first selective serotonin re-uptake inhibitor (SSRI) available for prescription.

First introduced in 1987, it quickly became the most widely prescribed antidepressant medication ever. In fact, sales of Prozac were $1.2 billion in 1995, and over 6 million Americans use it regularly. Prozac's success has spawned other SSRIs, including Zoloft (sertraline hydrochloride), Luvox (fluvoxamine), and Paxil (paroxetine hydrochloride). The SSRIs desensitize a receptor on the neuron that would normally absorb serotonin into the cell, allowing a greater supply of serotonin in the synapse. Serotonin is believed to be one of the brain's natural antidepressants, so higher serotonin levels enhance mood and bring about a reduction in anxiety and depressive symptoms. The reported side effects of Prozac include nausea, headaches, anxiety and nervousness, insomnia, drowsiness, diarrhea, dry mouth, loss of appetite, sweating, tremors, and rashes. The SSRIs also commonly reduce sex drive and may interfere with the ability to attain orgasm, especially in women.

Prozac is more likely than other antidepressants to cause restlessness and agitation. Zoloft and Paxil are similar to Prozac in terms of side effects. However, Paxil tends to be more sedating, making it preferable for people with anxiety or insomnia. Zoloft generally falls in between the stimulating Prozac and the sedating Paxil, but individuals differ in their responses. Luvox is most often used to treat obsessive-compulsive disorder.

My own clinical experience with these agents has been mixed. Most people have to choose between the antidepressant effect and the side effects—which are worse? In my experience, the vast majority of these patients can actually do better on natural supplements, which may have the same positive results, but without the side effects. The most useful of these have been kava and St. John's wort (see Chapter 12).

# The Other Antidepressants

The three antidepressants described here don't fall into the categories above.

## *Wellbutrin* (Bupropion hydrochloride)

Although it is not clear how this drug works, it appears to mildly inhibit the uptake of the neurotransmitters, serotonin, norepinephrine, and dopamine. Chemically related to the amphetamines, it usually has a more energizing effect than the other synthetic drugs. Side effects include seizures, restlessness, insomnia, irritability, and headaches.

## *Desyrel* (Trazodone hydrochloride)

Desyrel works on the serotonin system. Rather than being used for its antidepressant effects, it is most often prescribed along with Prozac because its sedating effect counteracts Prozac's tendency to produce insomnia. Desyrel's other side effects include headaches, upset stomach, low blood pressure, dizziness, and dry mouth. In men, it can cause a dangerous condition called *priapism*—painful, drug-induced erections that may not end upon discontinuing the drug. These side effects explain why Desyrel is seldom prescribed as an antidepressant.

## *Effexor* (Venlafaxine hydrochloride)

This medication inhibits serotonin re-uptake and boosts norepinephrine levels. Frequent side effects include nausea, dizziness, drowsiness, dry mouth, sleep disturbances, and increased blood pressure. When a patient is discontinuing use, because of its short half-life, dosages should be tapered off over two weeks to avoid withdrawal symptoms of severe rebound anxiety and depression. I have seen suicidal depression as a result of sudden Effexor withdrawal.

## *Serzone* (Venlafaxine hydrochloride)

The action of this medication is unclear; however, it is often recommended in cases of agitation, anxiety, and insomnia.

## Treating Drugs with Drugs

---

Since anxiety and insomnia are frequent side effects of many of these compounds, doctors will often add an antianxiety medication or a sedative. The practice of treating the side effects of one drug with another drug, with *its* own profile of side effects, is not the optimum approach, particularly with the other choices of treatments available. We will discuss this more in Chapter 9.

## Pharmaceuticals: Benzodiazepines

---

The most common antianxiety agents are the benzodiazepines—the best known being Valium. Almost 4 million Americans take these medications on a daily basis, often for years. Two-thirds of benzodiazepine prescriptions are written by family practitioners and internists, and most of the remainder by psychiatrists. Articles published in the late 1970s and early 1980s showed that when taken at the usually prescribed doses, dependence can occur after only one to two weeks.[1] With the increasing recognition of widespread abuse and dependency problems, the number of prescriptions for benzodiazepines gradually dropped from a high of 87 million in 1973 to 55 million in 1981.

This dip, however, was temporary, as a phenomenally aggressive marketing campaign for the introduction of Xanax in the late 1980s reversed the slide in popularity. With this new drug leading the way, prescriptions of all psychotropic medications, including benzodiazepines, again began to climb. Were people actually becoming more depressed and anxious, or were the drug companies simply doing a better job of selling? For an excellent examination of these issues, see Edward Drummond's *Overcoming Anxiety Without Tranquilizers*.[2]

## Side Effects

Although the benzodiazepines suppress the symptoms of anxiety for a few hours, they do not treat the underlying causes, and the anxiety returns as soon as the drug wears off. Moreover, there is a "rebound effect," occurring as a result of physical dependency, with the individual experiencing even worse symptoms than they started with. Often, *tolerance* will occur, meaning that even higher doses are needed for the same antianxiety effect. These factors—tolerance and withdrawal—describe an addiction that can be as difficult as heroin to break. A combination of physical and emotional dependency develops, and protection is not afforded by limiting to "occasional" use. Ignoring the warning that they are meant to be taken for only weeks at a time, overburdened doctors may continue to renew a prescription for many months or even years, sometimes simply over the phone.

### An Addictive Mix of Medications

#### Background

Jan was a 32-year-old secretary for an insurance company. She was married to an accountant, and they had a six-year-old daughter. Two years before I saw Jan, she had been in an auto accident, where another car hit her from behind with some force. She sustained a variety of injuries, including a shattered kneecap and whiplash, which left her with headaches and neck pain. The accident jarred her emotionally as well. During her weeklong hospital stay, she was given Valium as a muscle relaxant and antianxiety agent, and Restoril for sleep. The Restoril was understandable, as sleeping in a hospital can be difficult. In time, her injuries healed, but she was left with intermittent neck pain, relieved to some degree by Valium.

Jan was unable to end her dependence on Valium and Restoril. Her attempts to discontinue the medications were met with unbearable insomnia, followed by fatigue and inability to function. She was hooked, and her doctor continued to renew her prescriptions. She noticed herself becoming absent-minded; not remembering where she had put things in the house, forgetting appointments, and becoming increasingly tired and depressed. She had long since quit her job, unable to cope with any additional responsibilities. Life was bleak, and since the accident, she had a lingering fear of driving. She spent more and more time at home, doing less and less. Her concerned husband brought her to see a psychiatrist, who prescribed an antidepressant. Months later, with poor results from the antidepressant, she came to see me. I realized that she had the "benzodiazepine syndrome," and explained that her symptoms were due to the drugs themselves.

### Treatment

We began a program of psychotherapy and gradual withdrawal from the medication, both of which were successful. Unlike her previous attempts, this withdrawal was easier, and shorter than most because we used various supplements, particularly kava and valerian. These last two helped not only with the anxiety and insomnia, but the lingering neck pain as well. I also referred Jan to a chiropractor for help and body work. Jan was able to return to work, at a better job, and her husband thanked me for "giving me my wife back!"

---

Jan had most of the common side effects caused by benzodiazepines: impaired memory, confusion, depression, lack of coordination, and unwanted drowsiness. This daytime sedation and mental confusion can, like alcohol ingestion, lead to traffic accidents.[3] Another problem is *ataxia* or imbalance, which is especially problematic when it occurs in the elderly, where it can lead to falls, and often hip fractures.[4, 5]

As in Jan's case, chronic benzodiazepine use tends to maintain anxiety and promote depression, leading to social withdrawal and a narrowing of life focus. This may be a slow, insidious process, and no one may think to attribute it to the use of the drug. The resulting depression is often treated with antidepressants, rather than eliminating the source of the problem by stopping the benzodiazepine itself. This creates a vicious cycle with no escape for these unfortunate individuals.

Withdrawal effects from benzodiazepines include insomnia, anxiety, irritability, sweating, blurred vision, diarrhea, tremors, mental impairment, and headaches. Abrupt withdrawal from high doses can lead to seizures, or even death.[6] Fortunately, we have natural products like kava that can help with the transition off medication, although doctors' supervision is still essential.

## Treatment for Insomnia

The sleep induced by benzodiazepines is generally not restful and often produces a morning hangover. Benzodiazepines suppress REM or dream sleep, which is essential to mental health. For more information about the side effects and a full discussion of sleep disorders, see Chapter 9.

There are far better, more natural ways to enhance sleep, including relaxation techniques, diet, and exercise (see Chapter 9). There are also a host of natural remedies, including kava, which promote sleep without suppressing REM, and without a hangover. A 40-year-old male attorney who used kava before a big trial told me, "I had trouble getting to sleep last night, so I took two kava caps. Not only did they calm my circular thoughts—the ones that prevented me from falling asleep—but I awoke completely refreshed. I had the best sleep I've had in a long time!"

# Are Side Effects Inevitable?

The side effects of the antianxiety agents and antidepressants are due to the nature of synthetic drugs. When we affect one system in the body, we often affect others in both a positive and negative sense. It simply isn't possible to isolate the brain biochemically from the rest of the body. Medications may have a single intended action, but it is impossible for them not to affect other parts as well. This often creates unwanted, and sometimes dangerous, side effects (see *Talking Back to Prozac* by Peter Breggin and Edward Drummond's *Overcoming Anxiety without Tranquilizers,* mentioned previously).[7] Although it isn't common, I have seen severe toxic reactions to SSRIs, resulting in permanent damage to susceptible individuals.

It may seem odd that drugs can produce a side effect in some individuals but not in others. Yet each of us has a unique biochemical makeup. For reasons that are not totally understood, certain people respond better to one medication than another. They may have a more pronounced reduction in their depression, or they may not have any significant side effects. Another person could take the same dosage and have quite different results. Consequently, the physician's selection of the best antidepressant medication is often a matter of an educated guess, followed by trial and error.

For many people, particularly those who have come to me for a change to natural remedies, the side effects are so intense (as we saw with Jan), or the expense is so high, that they prefer to stop synthetic medications altogether. In many cases, antidepressants produce subtle emotional results as well—complaints of emotional flatness, dullness, of not caring. Replacing these with gentler herbs such as kava and/or St. John's wort allows a natural range of emotion and sharpness of mental functioning to emerge. They can also effectively treat the anxiety, depression, and insomnia, with minimal side effects. I have many patients who have made the switch. While the physical and psychological addiction made this difficult at first, the results were well worth it.

## Making the Right Decision

Despite the vast overuse of medication, it has an appropriate role in psychiatric treatment, as in cases of severe anxiety or depression, and bipolar disorder. The gentler actions of natural supplements are often more appropriate to resolve milder emotional imbalance and should be the first line of defense. Since they all have potentially harmful side effects, the more concentrated, targeted synthetic medications should be reserved for those instances when their benefits outweigh their costs. This is why a prescription is required from a psychiatrist or other medical practitioner. He or she is the one who can make an educated decision as to the best choice for you. Your role as the patient is to be a good observer and reporter, state your educated choices, and help guide the process. This is particularly important in view of my earlier comments about the negligence of some physicians regarding their prescribing habits. Be sure your doctor is not only competent, but that he or she listens to you and respects your input.

## The Pharmaceutical Industry and Mental Health

There was a strong movement in the 1970s and 1980s to limit the use of the benzodiazepines, but it ultimately failed. Barbara Gordon's book *I'm Dancing As Fast As I Can* documented her difficulties in dealing with her addiction.[8] Many respected doctors, journalists, and government officials spoke out about this abuse. The English physician Malcolm Lader put it well in his 1978 article, "Benzodiazepines: The Opium of the Masses," "It is much cheaper to tranquilize distraught housewives living in isolation in tower-blocks with nowhere for their children to play than to demolish these blocks and rebuild on a human scale, or even to provide play-groups. The drug industry, the government, the pharmacist, the taxpayer, and the doctor all have vested interests in medicalizing socially determined stress responses."[9]

Moreover, once out of medical school, a doctor's further professional "training" is virtually monopolized by the pharmaceutical industry. The industry funds university medical school-based research; finances "impartial" professional journals through its advertising; sponsors most medical conferences; and sends its representatives to visit physicians, dispensing samples along with the latest research. Already overloaded and short of time, doctors rely on these sources of information for their continuing education. This dilemma is compounded by doctors' lack of exposure to education about natural medicine during training. Doctors are taught a mechanistic view of the human organism and a technological approach to diagnosis and treatment.

In addition, mental health has become a stepchild of medicine, poorly reimbursed by insurers, despite the fact that good psychiatric care requires time—to listen, to interact, and to begin a healing alliance. Too often psychiatric visits are limited to brief "medication visits," and psychiatrists, like many other physicians, have become pill-pushers. The HMOs, Veteran's Administration, other government-funded medical care, and private insurers have all cut back on mental health services. A 1998 study by the Hay Institute found benefits had been cut 54% over the past 10 years. This has left many people with the choices of going untreated; taking ineffective, or even dangerous, medication from overburdened doctors; or taking charge of their own health care, paying out-of-pocket, and going the natural route.

# Mind, Body, and Nature:
# A Holistic Approach

Evidence is strong that this last option is growing by leaps and bounds. We believe that in the future we will see insurance company subsidization of integrated health care. This would take the best from Western and natural medicine, and pay for health maintenance, nutritional supplements, and the services of natural health practitioners. Successful programs will also include physician and consumer education in these methods, and will attend to the health of the whole person—mind, body, and spirit.

Years ago, when I began using a more natural approach in my practice, I was met with skepticism from my patients—until they saw the results. I was also met with outright disbelief from more conservative colleagues, who attributed my successes to "the placebo effect." For anyone who understands the mind-body continuum (and the growing science of psycho-neuro-immuno-endocrinology), the placebo effect is a major component in healing, not to be dismissed out of hand. Over the years, the results have spoken for themselves, and patients are increasingly referred specifically for a more holistic approach, including orthomolecular or nutritional treatment. Physicians are now looking twice at this "new medicine."

We have discussed how conventional medicine treats most illnesses symptomatically, most often with prescription drugs. It has become clear that these conditions reflect imbalances in our body chemistry and physiology, and can be treated more effectively with a natural approach. Plants, animals, and human beings are part of the continuum of nature and have evolved to interact together biochemically. This leads us to the discussion of herbs, nature's medicine.

# Advantages of Natural vs.
# Synthetic Substances

As we have seen, the antianxiety drugs have unwanted side effects, including sedation. They are also addictive, become ineffective over time, and are potentially lethal in overdose, especially when mixed with alcohol or barbiturates. By comparison, the natural antianxiety and antidepressant herbs have been used safely for thousands of years. They are non-addictive, less expensive, and have fewer and far less severe side effects. The multiple components in herbs are usually at a low enough concentration that they don't affect any one area too strongly. In fact, those extra effects are often *positive*, producing healing by means of the synergy of the combined components.

For millenia, herbs have been believed to promote balance and healing, rather than just to treat symptoms. Herbs such as kava, St. John's wort, ginseng, and valerian have been used successfully for thousands of years to treat the symptoms of anxiety, depression, and insomnia that are part of the stress cycle. We are just now rediscovering these gifts of nature, conducting research to prove their properties, and putting them to clinical use. I always prefer a natural remedy as my first resort.

# The Advantages of Kava

In cases of anxiety, my first choice is kava. It calms without sedating, and enhances awareness, concentration, and clarity of focus, all without serious side effects, lethal effects, or addictive potential. In higher doses, kava produces restful, restorative sleep. You will learn more about this remarkable South Pacific herb beginning in the next chapter.

## CHAPTER 6

# What Is Kava?

In this chapter, we introduce kava through a contemporary case example. We then explore its botany, history, and the role it has played in South Pacific culture over the centuries. We go on to trace the evolving interest of Westerners in kava, beginning with Captain Cook's arrival on the islands in the 1700s, and leading up to its present-day use.

Phil was a 44-year-old salesman who had been out of work for the first time in years. As he put it, "I was having trouble sleeping, and then flubbed a couple of job interviews. I have to admit, I was getting a little nervous. My buddy Tony told me about kava, and I figured what have I got to lose? I started using it. I can't recommend the taste, but my nerves got better, and I started sleeping again. Last week I went on an interview, and I felt like my old self. Happy ending—I got the job."

Too good to be true? Some might be inclined to dismiss Phil's story as "anecdotal," or at best, as an example of a "placebo effect" due to the belief that a substance will be effective. Yet accounts from individuals whose stress and anxiety problems have been helped by kava continue to pile up. And, as we will show in the following chapters, good clinical research validates these anecdotes.

# Herb of the Islands

The way of life of the South Pacific has come to symbolize heaven on earth to many Westerners—the ultimate escape from urban pressures. So it is worth noting that the use of kava is perhaps the primary natural and cultural thread that runs through Oceania—the islands stretching from Hawaii to New Zealand, including Fiji, Samoa, Tonga, the Marshall and Solomon Islands, Vanuatu, Papua New Guinea, and Tahiti. The scientific name for kava (or kava kava), is *Piper methysticum* (Latin for "intoxicating pepper"). This name refers to both the plant and the beverage prepared from its roots. Depending on the area of the Pacific, it has also been called *awa, waka, lawena,* or *yaqona.* Kava has been used for centuries medicinally, as well as for the preparation of a calming social and ceremonial drink. It remains an essential part of island life today.

The drink is notorious for its bitter taste. Novelist and travel writer Paul Theroux, in his book *The Happy Isles of Oceania,* described his experience this way, "I sat and clapped a little as he handed me the shell—and drank it down in a gulp—then handed the empty shell back and clapped again. It had a revolting taste. It was lukewarm, and it had the slightly medicinal flavor of mouthwash to which some mud had been added. There was nothing alcoholic in it, though there was a mild afterburn and a hint of licorice."[1] Though others mention a slight flavor of lilac or clove, straight kava can safely be described as an acquired taste.

The first effect after drinking kava is usually a slight numbing of the tongue or the back of the throat. Successive shells increase the effect until one reaches a state of being extremely relaxed—both physically and emotionally. But the kava experience is not done to shut out the world. Quite the opposite. Over and over again, kava enthusiasts tell you how it brings the world in.

## Botany

Kava thrives in humid, tropical climates with evenly distributed rainfall at elevations of 500 to 1,000 feet above sea level. Though considered swamp loving, it can grow in stony ground, both when cultivated and in the wild. A lush, leafy green plant, it grows densely to a height of about 7 to 8 feet, and sometimes as tall as 12 to 20 feet. The plant's leaves are heart-shaped, smooth, shiny, and green on both sides.

Planted in a manner similar to sugarcane, sections of stalks, usually cut from the young branches of an old bush, are laid in trenches of mud to sprout. The newly planted stem cuttings must be protected from direct sunlight and wind. Once sprouted, stalk sections are then planted in shallow trenches, where they continue to send up new shoots, growing perennially. Sprawling rootlike stems, alternately disappearing below and surfacing above the soil, may reach lengths of nine feet. At maturity, in five to seven years, the masses of roots are ready for preparation of the kava beverage.

Terry Willard, president of the Canadian Association of Herbal Practitioners, sees a resonance between a plant's form and its function. "With kava, the metaphor is 'bringing order and calming disjointedness. When you see the kava plant, the leaf and stem system look very disjointed, but when you dig under the system and see the root, which is what we use, it's very orderly."

Kava gardens and plantations are typically passed on through successive generations of islanders, and many kava patches have been tended by the same families for well over a century, rather like the vineyards of France and Italy. In Hawaii, where kava was once widely grown, but nearly disappeared after the coming of missionaries, farmers find ancient but still usable kava roots growing in long-forgotten native gardens.

Botanists believe that *Piper methysticum* is a descendant of wild kava, *Piper wichmannii,* a naturally occurring plant that is still sometimes used by islanders when cultivated kava is in short supply. However, cultivated kava is greatly preferred by nearly all societies that use it. Like many of the intensively cultivated root plants of the Pacific, kava has lost the ability to reproduce on its own, and has long been dependent on humanity for its survival. The incredible diversity of kava "cultivars," or specially cultivated plants, is no accident. Farmers carefully selected and bred specific kava varieties for different purposes, including medicinal, recreational, and ritual uses.

The wide number of varieties of kava under cultivation rivals corn, coffee, potatoes, and other favorite crops, and its wide distribution across the Pacific suggests that it has been under cultivation for at least 3,000 years. Remember, the plant itself is no longer able to reproduce. Yet kava has survived the invasion, colonization, religious conversion, and development of Oceania, as well as tourism, social upheaval, and political reform. This speaks volumes about its value to those people who have worked to preserve and improve it over the centuries. We have them to thank for the opportunity we now have to share in its benefits.

# History

Imagine for a moment that you're a Polynesian of 3,000 years ago, getting ready to set sail from your overcrowded home island toward the unknown realms over the eastern horizon. You may find a new island on which to settle, or you may not. Whatever the case, your survival hinges on the supplies you bring with you to your new home.

So what do you and your fellow colonists bring with you on the voyage in your tiny, oceangoing outrigger canoe? With space at a premium, most of these early explorers opted for a few clothes, fishing gear, tools made from stones and shells, chickens and perhaps a few pigs, a few food plants to cultivate, and kava. And when one takes inventory of the myriad of medicinal, social, and cultural uses kava has been put to over the centuries, it's easy to see why these daring, stone age sailors wouldn't leave home without it.

While this story may be speculative, it is certain that kava's use throughout the islands was well established when British explorer Captain James Cook made his first voyage to the area in 1768. It was Cook who first described for the Western world the ceremonial use of the intoxicating drink prepared from the kava plant. Credit for the first detailed description of the plant, however, was given to Johann Georg Forster in 1777. He is the one who gave the plant its Latin name.

"[Kava] . . . is made in the most disgustful manner that can be imagined, from the juice contained in the roots of a species of pepper-tree. This root is cut small, and the pieces chewed by several people, who spit the macerated mass into a bowl, where some water (milk) of coconuts is poured on it. They then strain it through a quantity of the fibres of coconuts, squeezing the chips, till all their juices mix with the coconut milk; and the whole liquor is decanted into another bowl. They swallow this nauseous stuff as fast as possible; and some old topers value themselves on being able to empty a great number of bowls. . . . The pepper plant is in high esteem with all the natives of these islands as a sign of peace; because getting drunk together implies good fellowship."[2]

Though Forster may not be a big kava booster, he does seem to grasp some of its meaning to the natives. The missionary William Ellis, apparently with a bit more of an ax to grind, wrote in 1828 of kava drinking in the Society Islands:

"They were sometimes engaged for several days together, drinking the spirit as it issued from the still, sinking into a state of indescribable wretchedness and often practicing the most ferocious barbarities. . . . Under the unrestrained influence of their intoxicating draught, in their appearance and their actions, they resemble demons more than human beings."[3]

Kava is not a spirit, and its preparation does not involve a still. You can't believe everything you read. More notable than the horror stories, though, are the surprising number of positive references to kava made by the Europeans who first came into contact with the substance.

"It gives a pleasant, warm and cheerful, but lazy feeling, sociable, though not hilarious or loquacious; the reason is not obscured."[4]

"The head is affected pleasantly; you feel friendly, not beer sentimental; . . . kava quiets the mind; the world gains no new color or rose tint; it fits in its place and in one easily understandable whole."[5]

It appears that, from earliest Western contact, one's response to kava has been, to a great extent, determined by one's own cultural biases. Later in this chapter, we will explore the cultural context within which kava use has evolved over the centuries, and we will examine in brief the context of kava in the West.


# Traditional Medicine

The *British-Herbal Pharmacopoeia* recognizes kava as an herb effective to combat urogenital inflammation, promote urination, and settle an upset stomach.[6] It also recognizes kava as a sedative, an antimicrobial, and an anti-spasmodic. In traditional medicine, kava is also used to relieve headaches, to control weight, to ease the symptoms of asthma, to treat tuberculosis and gonorrhea, and topically to treat fungal infections and to soothe insect bites and other skin irritations. As we will see later, some traditional uses have been borne out by research, and kava-based medicines look set to extend the versatile plant's reach far beyond the relief of stress and anxiety.

## Western Interest

During the mid-1800s, scientific researchers traced kava's relaxing properties to a group of resinous compounds called *kavalactones*. Found in the plant's root, these compounds relax muscles without blocking the nerve signals that keep the muscles tense. This may explain how kava reduces physical tension without numbing mental processes. Kava contains six major kavalactones, and while chemists can make some of these in the laboratory, the resulting drink has yet to produce the same effects as kava prepared from fresh rootstock. The efficacy of kava does not stem from a single substance, but rather from a mixture, a blend of several kavalactones that results in a synergistic physiological effect. We will go into the chemistry and pharmacology of kava in later chapters.

## Kava's Role in South Pacific Culture

Among the various island peoples, there are many different legends of the origin of kava, either through its discovery by man or by it being given to him from God. Such myths are important components of the oral history of indigenous peoples, and they tell us about much more than kava. The following Samoan legend summarizes man's relationship to the sun, sky, water, and earth as well as to the "Divine Being" and the life cycle:

"Long ago there was a custom that one day a year, one of the families of Fitiuta must sacrifice a daughter to the sun. On the day of the 'celebration of the sun' a daughter from the family of Matainaumati went to Samoa to be sacrificed. The girl's name was Ui. When the sun came for the girl, he saw that she was very beautiful and, instead of eating her, he decided to take her as his wife, and took the girl to live with him in the sky. After a time, she became pregnant and wanted to go home so that her first child could be born in her family's village.

"While journeying home, Ui had a miscarriage, and the fetus floated away upon the waters, where it was found by the hermit crab, the plover, and the shrike. By manipulating the fetus and breathing life into it, the animals created the first Samoan chief, Tagaloa Ui.

"After his creation Tagaloa Ui made a kilt for himself out of *ti* leaves and started to walk toward the village of Fitiuta. On his way, he walked through a grove of kava plants and discovered the house of the mortal Pava. Pava invited the chief to enter his house, and there the first kava ceremony involving mortal men was held.

"When Tagaloa Ui entered the house, he took a place at the end of the house (today the seat of honor), and Pava sat in the front of the house (the traditional place for talking chiefs), and began to prepare the kava. Pava chewed and spit the kava into a taro leaf which served as the kava bowl.

"While Pava was wringing the kava, his son, Fa'alafi, laughed and played near the bowl. Tagaloa Ui instructed Pava to make the boy sit down and be quiet, but nothing was done about the irreverent boy. After several unheeded warnings, Tagaloa Ui picked up a coconut frond, formed it into a knife, and cut Pava's son into two pieces. Then Tagaloa Ui said to Pava, 'This is the food for the kava. This is your part and this is mine.'

"Then Tagaloa Ui said, 'Let us have a new kava ceremony.' Tagaloa Ui told two of Pava's sons to go to the highest mountain, and bring down a wooden kava bowl, coconut cups, a hibiscus strainer, and a new kind of kava. These things were brought and a second kava ceremony was started. When the kava was ready, Tagaloa Ui said, 'Bring me my cup first.' Tagaloa Ui did not drink the kava, but poured it onto his piece of the dead son of Pava and then onto Pava's piece. Then he said, '*Soifua*' (life). The two parts came together, and the boy lived. Pava was so happy he clapped his hands. Pava drank his cup of kava, and Tagaloa Ui gave the following orders: 'Pava, do not let children stand and talk while kava is being prepared for high chiefs, for the things belonging to high chiefs are sacred.' "

A number of ritual details of the Samoan kava ceremony still practiced today seem to derive directly from this myth. They are:

- The seating arrangements
- Prohibitions against children, or any unauthorized, untitled persons attending the ceremony
- The solemn atmosphere that must prevail
- The proper equipment for the preparation and distribution of the kava
- The order of drinking
- The pouring of a bit of kava onto the mat
- The concept of food for the kava
- The use of the term "*Soifua*"
- The clapping of hands when the kava is ready
- The duty of "talking chiefs" to direct the kava ceremony[7]

The Oceanian-based culture evolved in different ways on different islands—producing huge statue-buildings on Easter Island and elaborate woven featherwork on bird-rich New Zealand. Similarly, kava use has varied throughout Oceania. Kava has functioned as a potent medicine for ailments, as a social drink for chiefs and noblemen, and as a ritual accompaniment to most important life events, including births, deaths, marriages, journeys, and even as a prelude to tribal wars. As the highest form of welcome, modern-day dignitaries are still offered—and accept—a ceremonial cup. In fact, Lyndon Johnson, Hillary Clinton, and Pope John Paul II have all imbibed kava on their visits to Fiji.

The drinking of kava imbues a person with the power to bless a building, a bridge, or a marriage. Among many in Fiji, kava remains the initial offering during any life crisis. It is also used in socialization, negotiation, commemoration, and celebration. Kava is also offered to ancestors when one wants to invoke the power of a taboo. As a demonstration of its power today, Asesela Ravuvu, professor of pacific studies at the University of the South Pacific in Fiji, tells of kava being offered to the gods to stop some rowdy boys from drinking alcohol. They never drank again, for fear of the taboo. If a taboo is broken, kava is offered immediately, for fear that guilt will haunt the person.

When kava is traded, the exchange is reciprocal, and balance is always the goal. A peacemaker will initiate a kava offering between individuals, families, or groups in conflict. Their ancestors are invoked, their bond is re-created, and the problems are erased. Kava is offered to invoke spirits of protection for travelers, for important requests, and in appreciation for requests granted.

Processing of kava involves pounding, chewing, grating, or grinding stumps and roots to break up the rootstock, allowing the kavalactones to be more readily released. It can be prepared by extracting the powdered root with cold water. However, more potent beverages are prepared either by using hot water, by first chewing the rootstock, or by extracting with alcohol.

During the 1700s a common method of kava preparation involved pounding the rootstock into small pieces, which were then chewed by men or women. Though women were not allowed to drink kava, young girls, preferably virgins, with healthy teeth and strong jaws were required to chew their elders' kava. In other cultures, young boys also performed this task. When the chewing was completed, the chewer put the mouthful of pulp into a large wooden bowl where it was then mixed with cold water. After thoroughly mixing the pulp, the beverage was strained and served.

Today, the root is seldom prepared by chewing, and probably only in rural villages. Many islanders opposed giving this up. Experience told them that it produced a stronger drink. In fact, saliva is not the crucial ingredient, but the act of chewing itself transforms the rootstock into tiny particles, releasing more of the resin, resulting in an emulsion that is more readily absorbed.

## Kava vs. Alcohol

Oceania is one of the few culture areas (North America being another) that had no alcoholic beverages at the time of its first significant contact with Europeans in the eighteenth century. Here, kava was the beverage of choice used both ritually and socially for its mind- and mood-altering properties. After drinking kava, islanders awake refreshed. This is in contrast with alcohol, which impairs central nervous system function and leads to morning hangover, as well as physiological damage from prolonged usage.

Kava is gentle and does not promote boisterous behavior or aggressiveness. At worst, overindulging can lead to loss of muscle control and a strong urge to sleep. Theroux had this to say on the subject: "No one ever went haywire and beat up his wife after bingeing on yanggona [kava]. No one ever staggered home from a night around the kava bowl and thrashed his children, or insulted his boss, or got tattooed, or committed rape. The usual effect after a giggly interval was the staggers and then complete paralysis."[8]

# The Fall and Rise of Kava

The decline of ceremonial kava drinking parallels the era of colonialism and cultural domination. The invasion of Oceania by Europeans and Americans is a sadly familiar one. The formerly independent islands found their political structures dominated by nations thousands of miles away, their resources stripped for the economic gains of others, and their local cultures belittled and suppressed.

To convert the natives toward their religion and away from indigenous tradition, Christian missionaries, who accompanied the warships and plantation owners, made eradication of kava drinking a major part of their program. They also objected to it because the traditional way of chewing the root before consumption was too gross for their fine sensibilities. Edicts banning kava drinking became the law of the land on many islands, and growing the plant was often forbidden as well.

Westerners were sadly successful in substituting alcohol over kava as the recreational beverage of choice. Alcoholism, health problems, and hostility fueled by liquor consumption replaced the calmness and sociability promoted by kava. As the old Hawaiian proverb puts it, "The man who drinks awa [kava] is still a man, but the man who drinks liquor becomes a beast." These efforts to suppress kava worked, at least temporarily. Across the Pacific, kava's open use was largely abandoned by the beginning of the twentieth century. In the former kava stronghold of Hawaii, kava drinking completely disappeared by 1948, and the rum-based "kava bowl" cocktails on sale at tourist bars in Waikiki actually contain no kava.

Now, though, the pendulum has swung back, and the return of kava goes hand in hand with the increased spirit of pride and independence among Pacific Islanders. The governments of Fiji, Vanuatu, and other Pacific island nations actively promote kava growing, for both domestic consumption and as an export crop. Even some Christian churches now promote kava as a safer, benign alternative to alcohol. Some churches on Pohnpei incorporate the root into their rituals of atonement, with islanders symbolically bringing kava roots as symbols of repentance.[9]

## Kava Use in Hawaii

Kava is also showing signs of a comeback in Hawaii. There, it is referred to as "awa," pronounced "ava." Hawaiian nationalists promote it as a key component of their lost heritage, while small farmers see kava as a sustainable crop of high value and ideally suited to local conditions. Some technologically savvy Hawaiian kava growers are even marketing their products to mainland enthusiasts via the World Wide Web—a suitably modern setting for this ancient root.

## Kava Drinking in the South Pacific Today

Though perhaps less so in the most Western-influenced villages or towns, kava drinking today is still a kind of ceremony. It occurs at a special time, usually taking place at sundown after a hard day of work. In contrast to the American "happy hour," which is a fairly boisterous time to unwind over alcohol, kava drinkers partake in peace and quiet. Islanders refer to "listening to kava," a condition of pleasurable contemplation. Though no longer universally so, in many villages, only men are allowed to participate. The traditional taboo held that women drinking kava might weaken its power. But this perception is changing.

In the island nation of Vanuatu, most towns and villages have one or more *nakamals,* or "kava bars." A nakamal's facilities might range from a fancy western-style bar or lounge, to a hut or lean-to with a dirt floor. In the nakamal, the pounded,

strained kava liquid is served in a large bowl. Social status determines who gets to drink first. The coconut shell is filled
and down the hatch it goes. You often hear kava measured in
"shells" as in "I had five shells of the stuff." Occasionally, the
coconut shell is shared among the group. (More than one
travel book advises tourists to bring their own shell, to avoid
hepatitis!) Chris Kilham has some wonderful accounts of
"nakamal nights" in his book *Medicine Hunting in Paradise*.

In the next few chapters, we will discuss uses of kava,
what it does, how it works, how to take it, and the considerable research (primarily European) that validates and explains its valuable properties.

## CHAPTER 7

# Chemistry and Actions

N ow we will address the unique and complex chemistry of kava, and how these compounds act on the body in many different ways. This chapter contains some scientific information that may interest a professional more than a layperson. However, the information will help you understand the material in later chapters.

Dried kava contains many ingredients: starch, fibers, sugars, proteins, and minerals. Although a small amount of research has been conducted on the water-soluble component of the rootstock, the majority of the research has been done on the resin, which contains most, if not all, of the active, fat soluble components. These are the kavapyrones or kavalactones (a *lactone* is an organic compound containing oxygen), which typically make up anywhere from 3% to 20% of kava's dried weight. Other compounds include alkaloids (two from the roots and one, piper methystin, from the leaves), flavokavins, an alcohol, a phytosterol, ketones, and organic acids. The concentration of kavalactones is generally highest in the lateral roots (15%) and decreases progressively toward the aerial part of the plant (10% in the stump; 5% in the basal stems).[1]

# Extraction Process

During the 1700s, a common method of kava preparation involved pounding the rootstock into small pieces, which were then chewed. When the chewing was completed, the chewer put the mouthful of pulp into a large wooden bowl where it was then mixed with cold water, strained, and served, as described in Chapter 6. The other traditional method of preparation was manually grinding and pounding the root, then adding water. The chewing method seems to produce the more potent kava drink. The reason for this was once thought to be related to the enzymes contained in saliva.

In 1939, researcher A.G. Van Veen discovered that for kava to be most effective, the rootstock must be emulsified to disperse the ingredients—in water, saliva, lecithin, or oil.[2, 3] It is now accepted that the lipid soluble material is released into aqueous solution through emulsification and that this process is mechanical rather than enzymatic or chemical. Present-day technological extraction methods take this into account. The kava roots destined for export are carefully washed, cut up, and dried before being mechanically ground into a fine powder. The powder is then ready for mixing with water for drinking in the traditional way, or for extraction and processing.

# Whole Kava vs. Extracted
# or Synthesized "Active Ingredients"

When confronted with a plant that exhibits healing properties, conventional medicine's response is often to break it down chemically in search of an elusive "active ingredient" that can be extracted or synthesized, and hopefully, patented. But in the case of kava, as with so many other healing herbs, this ignores the power of the whole. Vincent Lebot deserves to be quoted at length on the subject: "Kavalactones can now be synthesized, but these synthetics do not induce the same physiological effects as the natural extract. The efficacy of kava does not stem from a single substance but rather from a mixture, a blend of several kavalactones, that results in a synergistic physiological effect. Each kavalactone so depends on the presence of the others that unaltered extracts produce more psychoactive results than does any single isolated substance."[4] One study suggested that the human brain absorbs the lactones in whole kava much more readily than it does in the form of isolated kavalactones.[5]

With St. John's wort, for example, it was once thought that the active psychoactive ingredient was hypericin, and that its main mode of action was MAO inhibition. Later research proved both ideas to be less conclusive, with the activity stemming from a synergistic action among its various compounds and possibly from some other as-yet undiscovered ingredient and mode of action. Similarly, kavalactones may simply be markers for the as-yet undiscovered "real thing." Meanwhile, the different compounds affect different target cells and symptoms, maximizing healing effects while minimizing side effects. Just as hypericin as a marker for St. John's wort reflects only a small aspect of the herb's antidepressant and anti-anxiety qualities, so it is with kava. For maximum effectiveness, standardization must be multifaceted, addressing the potency, activity, species, and part of the plant used.

We have available highly sophisticated means of determining the kavalactone profile.[6] You might wonder if the wide variety of kava under cultivation (or "cultivars") produces problems in standardizing the product that shows up on North American and European shelves. According to Steven Dentali, a respected consultant to the herbal industry

## Components of Kava

In 1973, pharmacologist Alexander Shulgin divided the kava components into three categories: major (dihydrokavain, kavain, and methysticin), minor (yangonin, dihydromethysticin, desmethoxyyangonin, flavokavin A, pinostrobinchalcone, dihydrotecto-chrysin, aplinetinchalcone, aplinetin, and dihydro-oroxylin A), and trace (11-methoxy-nor-yangonin, 11-methoxyyangonin, and flavokavin B). In these last two categories are flavokavins that may be the source of the yellow skin condition discoloration seen in chronic kava users.[7]

Vincent Lebot later categorized six major kava-lactones (kavain, dihydrokavain, yangonin, dimethoxy-yangonin, methysticin, and dihydromethysticin) and nine minor ones, all pharmacologically active. The proportions of these kavalactones vary widely in the different cultivars grown for human consumption, creating a unique "cocktail" for each cultivar.[8] Content is also affected by such factors as the age of the plant and specific environmental factors, such as where and how it is grown, the soil conditions, climate, harvesting, drying, and processing methods. Although they were ignorant of modern chemistry and genetics, the Pacific Islanders who first domesticated kava cultivated different varieties for specific purposes, exemplifying an interesting interaction between the human and plant worlds.

and author of a major safety review of kava, "There is no problem in standardizing for total kavalactone (or more accurately, kavapyrone) content, although the relative concentration of individual kavapyrones may vary. The total amount of kava-

Some kava varieties were meant for everyday use by the common folk, and others were reserved for high-ranking chiefs and princes or were used only for special ceremonies. Some were particularly mild, while one type, "two-day kava," was notorious for its potency and long-lasting effects. For the best psychoactive effect, high kavain and low dihydromethysticin is preferred, since kavain and dihydrokavain pass the blood-brain barrier most easily. That is, they are absorbed more readily from the bloodstream into the brain.

Kavain and dihydroyangonin predominate in the rootstalk, while dihydrokavain and dihydromethysticin, predominate in the stalks and leaves. Animal studies have shown that dihydromethysticin and dihydrokavain have sleep inducing, anticonvulsant, and muscle-relaxant properties. Some herbal companies are marketing kava extracts made from the above-ground portions of the plant, claiming that the leaf and stem-based products can deliver kava's muscle relaxing effects without producing intoxication. On the other hand, these components are similar to those found in *Piper methysticum's* wild cousin, *Piper wichamanii,* and both are often associated with nausea and headaches.

Because of the variability in kavalactone composition and overall activity, testing with high-performance liquid chromatography (HPLC) or at least, thin layer chromatography (TLC), is important to ensure the quality of the material sold as bulk herb or finished product.[9, 10]

pyrones in unprocessed underground material is reported to range between 5 and 15%, so standardization can be a matter of making a concentrated extract and ensuring that the finished material meets the desired specifications."

# How Does It Work?

Much research on the basics of kava chemistry and how it acts on a living body has already been done. Many of these studies have used laboratory animals, a subject that may be troubling for some. So, without passing judgment on the ethics of the tests themselves, following are some of the findings.

## Actions on the Nervous System

Kavalactones have been shown to relieve anxiety and pain and to relax muscles in laboratory animals. An underlying question is the seeming paradox of its actions; it relaxes without sedating at lower doses, while higher doses sedate but in a different way from other known sedatives.

## Antianxiety Effects

Early studies suggested that kava affects the nervous system through a reduction of activity in the spinal part of the nervous system rather than in the higher centers of the brain.[11] Later studies show that the limbic system, or emotional center, is also involved. Understanding this effect calls for a brief lesson in brain anatomy and function.

The central nervous system is comprised of the brain, the spinal cord of nerves that carry messages to and from the brain, and the peripheral nerves that connect these to various parts of the body. The brain itself may be divided into three parts based on levels of evolution. The newest part, in evolutionary terms, is the *neocortical part,* the site of higher thought functions. Next is the *limbic system,* the emotional control center—which contains the following:

- The pituitary or master gland
- The amygdala, which is the center for registering fear and anger

• The hypothalamus, which mediates the stress response as discussed in Chapter 2

Last is the most primitive level—comprised of the brain stem and reticular formation—which joins the brain to the spinal cord. This is the auto-pilot of the brain, governing the basic vital functions such as breathing, heart rate, and digestion.

The effects of drugs on the nervous system will vary according to the target areas. The question is: Where and how does kava work on the nervous system? We do have some idea, although more research is needed for a complete understanding. Besides this anatomical map, we also know that the chemical messengers of the brain—such as neurotransmitters, endorphins, and neurohormones—act in many different locations of the brain and the body (for details, see Candace Pert's *Molecules of Emotion*).[12] As in many other fields, the current move is toward a "systems" rather than "linear" way of observation and analysis. All that said, anatomically based research has given us a great deal of valuable information.

Kava appears to work on the body and brain in a manner different from all known pharmaceuticals that produce sedation and muscle relaxation. For one, kava does not appear to bind to the brain's opiate receptors, meaning that it reduces pain in a manner unrelated to that of morphine and other opiates, or even aspirin. Nor are these pain-relieving effects due to its sedating and muscle-relaxing effects.[13]

A 1991 EEG study showed that kava acted on the limbic system and primarily on the *amygdala,* the seat of the emotions. This may explain how it can promote sleep even in the absence of sedation. This would also explain the pleasant feelings associated with its use, as feelings of fear and anger are subdued.[14]

## Effects on GABA, the "Valium" Receptor

GABA, or gamma-aminobutyric acid, is a naturally occurring, calming amino acid. Its plentiful receptors in the brain are the site of action of the benzodiazepines. We might expect that since the actions of kava are similar to the benzodiazepines, it would bind to these receptors. Earlier animal studies, however, indicated that kavalactones bind only weakly, if at all, to these receptors.[15]

Later research shows that kavapyrones do mediate sedative effects by way of GABA-receptor binding, with the hippocampus and amygdala showing the highest levels of enhancement. These effects were due to an increase in the *number* of GABA binding sites rather than to a change in *affinity*. The authors also observed that when kava was mixed with a barbiturate, kava potentiated its sedating effects. They suggest that the previous study might have seen little effect on GABA's binding activity for a number of reasons, including: 1) the previous authors looked at areas atypical for kavapyrone effect (frontal cortex and cerebellum) as opposed to the usual target brain centers for its actions (hippocampus, amygdala, and medulla oblongata); 2) only two kavapyrone concentrations (100 M and 1 mm) were used; 3) investigators used pure compounds of methysticin, dihydromethysticin, kavain, and dihydrokavain rather than a whole extract which more closely estimates its pharmacological effect in vivo. [16]

## Muscle-Relaxing, Analgesic, and Anticonvulsant Effects

The kavalactones are non-sedating muscle relaxants. Moreover, these effects are on both skeletal (striated, voluntary) muscle and smooth or involuntary muscle, such as that of the heart, lungs, and digestive system.

Kavalactones also have strong anticonvulsant effects, as seen in studies of rats pretreated with strychnine, which caused them to convulse. In addition, muscle contractions in isolated smooth muscle in rats also were inhibited by the pyrones. Its analgesic effect is superior to aspirin's, but less marked than that of morphine. [17, 18]

In a significant 1982 study, Y.N. Singh studied the effects of kava in the muscles and nerve tissue of mice and frogs.[19] His study found that kava differed from other antianxiety drugs by causing a direct action on muscle contractibility, instead of by inhibiting neuromuscular transmission. This makes kava more closely related to local anesthetics in its physiological effects (as anyone who's ever tasted the stuff can attest), and helps explain why very high doses can cause ataxia and temporary paralysis in the lower limbs without loss in consciousness. This, however, was an "in vitro" study; that is, done on a tissue preparation, which doesn't mean it is necessarily a muscle relaxant when taken orally.

Kavain substantially inhibited the contractile response in guinea pig ileum (gut) tissues, further confirming kava's relaxant properties on smooth muscle, i.e., the "involuntary" muscles of the gut, heart, and other organs. However, the kavain had no effect on the ileum strips which were subjected to caffeine-induced contractions. The final results suggest that kavain may act in a non-specific way on the smooth muscle membrane. Also, a potential antipathy between kavain and caffeine is suggested. This might mean that you should avoid caffeine if you want to enjoy the full relaxant effects of kava. On the other hand, such conclusions may be stretching it—from caffeine-treated ilium to oral kava and java is a long way.[20]

Kavalactones inhibit convulsions caused by strychnine, electroshock, and pentylenetetrazole in animals. Here, as in other studies, the authors note that multiple constituents of *Piper methysticum* have an additive or synergistic effect compared to the individual kavalactones. Peripherally, kavalactones also produce local anesthesia similar to that of procaine. The analgesia of kava is not reversed by "naloxone," a chemical that blocks the action of narcotics. This indicates that the mode of action of kava's pain-killing effects differs from that of the narcotics, such as morphine.[21]

A 1995 rat brain study provides further clues as to the physical mechanisms of kava's relaxation effects. It showed that kavain affects transmission of electrical impulse conduction by inhibition of voltage-dependent sodium channels, a common target of anti-epileptic drugs.[22]

The influence of kavain on veratridine-stimulated increases in intrasynaptasomal Na+ concentrations of rat cerebrocortical synaptosomes was investigated.

A recent report suggests that kavain and/or methysticin suppress release of the excitatory amino acid neurotransmitter glutamate, leading to a calming effect.[23]

Similar to the anticonvulsant drug memantine, in rodent experiments, methysticin and dihydromethysticin protected the brain cells against damage due to lack of blood supply. It had a similar protective effect on test-tube tissue preparations deprived of oxygen. The effect appears to be by direct action on the neurons.[24] Not surprisingly, the effectiveness of whole root extracts appears to be greater than that of isolated kavalactones.[25] A 1988 study also found that the kava resin was more effective in animal studies than the individual constituents.[26]

# Conclusion

Science has far more to learn about the mechanisms of kava's action. One consistent finding is that kava worked best as a whole extract. These discoveries in turn may shed new light on the complex interactions between the human body and brain, and afford new, less toxic opportunities for healing. Kava is a safe, effective, and natural treatment for stress, anxiety, and insomnia, as well as a host of other physical and psychological ailments. In the next chapter, we will describe kava's clinical uses and the research that backs it up.

## CHAPTER 8

# Clinical Uses of Kava

People want to know 'what is kava good for?'
Plants don't come with instructions.
We must learn from them what they're for.

—*Steven Dentali, Ph.D., associate editor,* Medical Herbalism

## What Does Kava Do?

What role can kava play in treating stress and anxiety?
Here's what Kristen, a 29-year-old journalist from Arizona,
had to say.

### Background

"I've been taking kava off and on for years, as a sleep aid
and nerve tonic. I am a fairly high-strung person. Throughout my life, I've been diagnosed with depression a bunch of
times. Last year, I hit a very low period, and I finally found

a doctor with some integrity, who took the time to find out what caused my depression. Then it all made sense. She told me I seemed to have anxiety-induced depression. I stress, I get irritable and stress even more, and that taxes my brain and produces some kind of chemical response, and bam! I'm hit with a nasty depression that I can't drag myself out of.

"Years ago, before this happened, I went through a phase (also right before a depressive period) where I was having regular panic attacks. These weren't just bouts of anxiety, but actual clinical panic attacks. I'd hyperventilate, become absolutely convinced that I was dying, having a stroke, or a having heart attack—you name it. I was the editor of the college newspaper then, and it was rather embarrassing, to say the least, when one of these attacks would hit me. I'd be sitting in my office wondering if I should (or could) go ask a reporter to take me to the hospital. Twice, I actually did ask someone, and he walked me outside. I would eventually calm down.

### Using Kava

"Right after that, I asked a friend who was training as an herbalist to recommend an herb for 'brain function.' She gave me kava, and I took it for about a month, three times a day. I don't know that it improved my brain function, exactly, but I noticed during that time that I was much easier to get along with. I slept better, I wasn't so high-strung, and everything came easier.

"I don't use it all the time anymore, but it's helped me when I couldn't sleep because I was simply too stressed, lying in bed trying to balance bills and paychecks. On those days when my mind is racing and I'm fretting needlessly about money, school, work, romance, or whatever, I take two dropperfuls of kava and boom—I'm relaxed.

"I'm amazed at how it has improved my life. I don't get that circular thinking, and it makes it easier for me to step back and look at everything calmly. So I've got only $10 in my bank account, and I don't know what I'm going to do with my life? Oh well! The sky is falling? Just give me some kava so I can watch it happen, with no panic."

———————

This is quite a story! Kristen had a variety of problems over time: depression, panic attacks, insomnia, and a stressed, racing mind. The solution for all of them has been kava. She sounds like the kava poster child! Is this too good to be true?

According to a large body of scientific research, along with reports from other health practitioners and my own clinical experience, Kristen's case is not an isolated one.

## European Use of Herbal Medicine

Kava has a history of use in Europe—particularly France, Switzerland, and Germany. Most of the research has been done in Germany and some in Australia, because of its proximity to Oceania. Do you wonder why the United States has not been open to the practice of herbal medicine until recently? Despite a rich heritage of information, from both European and Native American sources, the legacy was lost in the early part of the 1900s. Phytomedicine (plant-based medicine) was removed from medical school curriculums, and replaced by technological medicine and pharmaceuticals. Meanwhile, in some European countries, natural medicine continued to be taught alongside Western medicine, giving the Europeans a clear advantage in knowledge and research opportunities. It is only now that we have begun to revisit this cornucopia of healing resources.

In Germany, where doctors can prescribe herbal as well as synthetic products, they frequently choose the more benign, and often more effective, plant materials. Herbs containing chemical substances similar to our own, work as natural synergistic groups of compounds. Like food, these gifts of nature are available to nurture and heal us. Most of our pharmaceuticals are actually plant-based, just modified and refined for more specific actions and for patentability, since there is no return on their research investment otherwise. These changes are not always for the best, however, since concentrating a substance often removes its protective compounds and increases the possibility of side effects.

A good example of the drug/herb comparison is St. John's wort, which appears to work as well as the synthetic antidepressants for mild to moderate depression, but without their often intolerable side effects. In Germany, physicians prescribe it anywhere from 10 to 20 times more often than Prozac (see Chapter 5). Now that the American population is becoming more educated and is no longer willing to accept the shortcomings of conventional medicine, our medical community is finally beginning to catch on. The National Institutes of Health are funding a $4.3 million study at Duke University School of Medicine on the use of St. John's wort for severe depression. The movement toward complementary or integrated medicine has been well launched, with 63 medical schools currently teaching courses in alternative medicine. These projects are harbingers of things to come.

## German Commission E Monograph

The German Commission E is an expert advisory panel to the German equivalent of the U.S. Food and Drug Administration (FDA). They review the available literature on various herbs, to determine their suitability as non-prescription medicines. Commission E has published nearly 400 monographs evaluating herbal medicines as to their effectiveness, side effects, dosage, interactions with conventional medicines, and contraindications. An English translation by an elite team of herbal specialists, headed by Mark Blumenthal and Joerg Gruenwald, is newly available through the American Botanical Council. With translation and commentary, it will be one of the most reliable sources of information on the use of herbal products, especially for health professionals (see Appendix B).

# Stress and Anxiety

If we are looking for analogies with conventional drugs, and consider St. John's wort to be "Nature's Prozac," then kava is "Nature's Valium." But unlike users of Valium and other antianxiety drugs, the mind of the kava user remains clear, with many even reporting a sharpening of physical coordination and mental clarity. Research bears out these findings, as does clinical experience.

### How Kava Helps Anxiety

A screenwriter patient of mine took a dose of kava (40 drops of tincture) to calm his nerves before an initial meeting with a group of studio executives. By his report, not only did his anxiety disappear, but he was able to present his material and think on his feet more clearly than ever.

Forty-seven-year-old Jessica uses kava when she is overwhelmed with work schedules and deadlines. She states, "Kava doesn't overpower you. It relaxes your muscles and calms your emotions without changing your personality. You're still yourself, just not as tense or anxious."

Jessica's observation is echoed by Wayne Silverman of the American Botanical Council, "People are interested in the subtlety of kava. That makes kava more palatable than many of the conventional medications."

## Commission E Monograph Summary for Kava

The Commission E kava monograph is summarized below:

**Uses:** Conditions of nervous anxiety, stress, and restlessness (translated by Gruenwald), or nervous anxiety, tension, and agitation (translated by Schulz, 1997). *Author's Note:* The subtle differences in meaning—"stress" versus "tension" and "agitation" versus "restlessness" have implications, since almost all research to date is in German, and our knowledge is based on the translator's interpretation. There are also significant cultural differences between the United States and Germany. We need U.S.-based research in order to really understand the spectrum of use and the effects of a substance, especially when the measures are as subjective as emotional states and responses.

**Contraindications:** Pregnancy, nursing, and endogenous depression.

**Side Effects:** Extended intake can cause a temporary yellow discoloration of the skin, hair, and nails. In this case, further applications of this drug must be discontinued. In rare cases, allergic skin reactions can occur. Accommodative disturbances, such as

# Clinical Studies

What does the research show about the effectiveness of kava in reducing anxiety? There have been six double-blind studies of kava in patients with anxiety. "Double blind" means that neither the participants nor the doctors know who is getting the active compound, in this case, kava, or an inactive "dummy" pill.

enlargement of the pupils and disturbances of oculomotor equilibrium, have also been described (see Chapter 11).

**Interactions with Other Drugs:** Potentiation of effectiveness is possible for substances acting on the central nervous system, such as alcohol, barbiturates, and psychopharmacological agents (see Chapter 11).

**Dosage:** Equivalent of 60 to 120 kava pyrones (kavalactones).

**Mode of Administration:** Comminuted rhizome and other galenic preparations for oral use. This means that the root and extract can be taken in oral preparations.

**Duration of Application:** Not more than three months without medical advice. *Author's Note:* Even when administered within its prescribed dosages, this herb may adversely affect motor reflexes and judgment for driving and/or operating heavy machinery.

**Action:** Antianxiety. In animal experiments, a potentiation of narcosis (sedation), anticonvulsive, antispasmodic, and central muscular relaxant effects were described.

### Kava vs. Placebo

Volz's 1997 double-blind placebo-controlled study represents a major step forward in kava research. It lasted 25 weeks and had 101 participants, making it a longer and larger study than any previous study on the effects of kava on anxiety disorder. The dose was one capsule of WS1490 extract (Schwabe), containing 70 mg kavalactones, taken three times daily.

Subjects had to have at least one of the following diagnoses by DSM-III-R criteria: agoraphobia, social phobia, generalized anxiety disorder, or adaptation disorder. The criteria for inclusion were consistent with U.S. standards, since the DSM-III-R is the official diagnostic manual used by the American Psychiatric Association. The Hamilton Anxiety Scale (HAMA) was used by the examining physicians to measure the severity of symptoms, with a score over 18—indicating moderate to severe anxiety—necessary for inclusion in the study. A 90-item Self-Report Symptom Inventory was also used so that the participants could rate their subjective experience.

After eight weeks, and continuing through the rest of the study, the kava group showed a significant improvement compared to the placebo group, on both physician-rated and self-rated scales. They also showed fewer side effects. In fact, the inert "placebo" pill produced more side effects than the real one. While placebo treatment almost always causes side effects, these extra side effects were most likely the results of their already-existing and untreated anxiety. Side effects in the kava group were few and minor, and laboratory tests showed no abnormal changes.

In summary, Volz's study showed that anxiety and depression significantly decreased, as did physical symptoms, including headaches, breathlessness, heart palpitations, chest or stomach pains, and faintness.[1] Interestingly, a similar 1996 study with 58 subjects using the same product showed that, unlike the previous study, kava worked better than the placebo from the outset. A majority of the kava users improved markedly after one week, with the improvement continuing through week four, which was the end of the survey period. The placebo group showed little change in their anxiety levels.[2]

Possible explanations for this difference in the onset of the effects of kava (week one vs. week eight) compared to placebo are as follows:

1. The Volz group were more seriously ill to start with, having an average illness duration of 6.5 months, and many had more than one diagnosis, including depression, making them more difficult to treat.

2. The placebo effect in the Volz group was particularly high, thereby decreasing the gap in results between the two groups.

Similarly rapid results were seen in two other randomized, placebo-controlled double-blind studies that followed 40 women with menopause-related anxiety symptoms. Subjects had improvement in symptoms after one week, reaching optimal levels at four weeks, and maintaining this comparative benefit for the full eight weeks of the study.[3, 4]

A 1989 study determined that an extract of kavain produced emotional and muscular relaxation while simultaneously stimulating the thinking process and activity. This study shows that an isolated compound, kavain, extract of kava, can also have a positive result. In general, though, research indicates that the whole extract is superior to the isolated compounds.[5] (See Chapter 7.)

### Kava vs. Benzodiazepines

In several studies, we've seen that kava produces positive effects when compared to a placebo. That tells us it's better than nothing. But the question remains: How does it compare to the most widely prescribed pharmaceuticals—the benzodiazepines (see Chapter 5)? The following studies attempted to provide answers in terms of both efficacy and safety. As you already know, medications such as Valium, Xanax, and Klonopin have the potential to relieve anxiety and insomnia, but with potent side effects, including dependency and addiction.

A 1993 study of 12 volunteers compared the effects on mental function of a standardized kava extract (WS 1490,

70 mg, three times a day) versus oxazepam (Serax). The 12 volunteers were tested on word recognition, measured in terms of accuracy, reaction time, and EEG responses. First, the oxazepam group "showed significant changes toward a less active, more introverted and drowsy behavior," while the kava group showed no such tendency. More importantly, oxazepam decreased both the speed of reaction time and the quality of recognition responses. Kava, on the other hand, *improved* reaction time and *enhanced* recognition. The researchers concluded that these results indicate "enhanced memory performance under kava . . . and a greatly impaired performance [with] oxazepam." This seems to confirm the claim that kava, as opposed to benzodiazepines, does not sedate. Moreover, rather than impairing mental sharpness, it actually improves it. This study was only comparing mental function and physical reaction time. What about relaxation? In two other studies, kava compares very favorably to two popular benzodiazepines in terms of relieving anxiety—but without the drugs' side effects.[6]

Another 1993 double-blind study followed 174 patients with anxiety symptoms for a period of six weeks. Patients received either 15 mg of oxazepam (Serax), 9 mg of bromazepam (a European benzodiazepine), or 300 mg of a 70% kavalactone extract daily. Kava matched both drug groups in improving anxiety scores as measured by the Hamilton Anxiety Scale (HAMA).[7]

In a 1990 study of 38 outpatients, half were treated with oxazepam, and half with kavain (a single kavalactone). Kavain relieved anxiety just as well as the pharmaceutical, and with no adverse effects.[8]

## Conclusions

Since German diagnostic criteria differ, some of these studies have been criticized for not using more precise criteria. We may also lose something in language and cultural translation. However, in the largest, longest-running study to date, Volz used the DSM-III-R (American-based) diagnostic categories. All the studies described here show that the participants gained some relief from their suffering and that kava compared well to benzodiazepines, without the latter's adverse effects. In studies where it was measured, kava actually enhanced mental functioning. These results look quite promising. Does kava lose its touch when it crosses the Atlantic? Only American research will tell.

## Muscle-Relaxing, Analgesic, and Anticonvulsant Effects

"By far the best use for kava is as a muscle relaxant," says Terry Willard, president of the Canadian Association of Herbal Practitioners. "Some researchers have suggested that kava in high doses impairs coordination, but we've found that in lower doses it actually enhances physical dexterity. We use kava in treating professional athletes, which up here (Calgary) mainly means hockey players. They say it not only handles their muscle tension, but it "slows the action down," and improves eye-hand coordination. It also calms their minds and gives them greater clarity. The ones who've tried it swear by it."

Willard's observation makes sense. Most stress-reduction techniques take advantage of the fact that it is practically impossible to be anxious when you are physically relaxed. In my own practice, when patients are able to simply release their physical tension, they become more present and more able to listen and take things in around them. Jodi, a stressed-out secretary, with chronic neck and shoulder tension, swears by a dose of 40 drops of kava tincture before a therapeutic massage. Not only is she more relaxed going in, but she says she gets more benefit from her massage session.

Singh's 1983 *in vitro* study (i.e., in a test tube) demonstrated that rather than sedating the central nervous system, the kavalactones have a distinctive direct muscle-relaxing effect (see Chapter 7). This makes kava useful for the treatment of nervous tension and conditions associated with skeletal muscle spasm and tension such as headaches caused by neck tension.[9]

The analgesic activities of kava resin and kavalactones have been demonstrated in several studies covered in Chapter 7. In brief, kava has a unique analgesic action. It differs in action from the opiates, such as morphine and codeine, and may work in some ways like the local anesthetic procaine. In one study, it was shown to enhance the pain-relieving qualities of aspirin.[10]

# Insomnia

Insomnia affects 43% of the population, and the incidence increases with age. Because of its seriousness, its impact on so many lives, and the benefits of kava in its treatment, we have devoted the next chapter specifically to sleep and insomnia. Following is a brief look at contemporary clinical use.

The earliest European explorers noted kava's sleep-inducing properties. More interesting than kava's ability to induce sleep is that it appears to improve the quality of sleep. Pacific Islanders often drink kava during periods when they have to subsist on fewer hours of sleep, and wish to get the most out of the sleep they do get. Explorer James Morrison noted in 1791 that after kava drinkers awake, "they are as fresh as if nothing had happened."[11]

Mark Blumenthal, director of the American Botanical Council, who pushes himself through a multiple time-zone travel schedule, often relies on kava to get him through the night. The energetic Blumenthal says, "I take two or three squirts of liquid kava tincture before bed, and because it helps me get a healthy dose of REM sleep, even when I don't get the recommended hours, I still wake up refreshed." Having spent time with Mark at many conferences, I can tell you that his keen mind and ready wit attest to the fact he's doing something right.[12]

Kava is especially useful since insomnia is almost always complicated by other factors, as with Jerry, a 40-year-old attorney, recovering from a recent auto accident. He wrote me the following note:

"I was in extreme pain from whiplash, and my orthopedic doctor prescribed everything under the sun ending in 'pam'—diazepam, lorazepam, oxazepam—to allow me a night of undisturbed sleep. Just getting to sleep was half the battle because of the pain. These pills would take a long time to work, and I'd have a hangover the next morning. I also couldn't take them at all during the day because they made me sleepy. I even tried some pain killers, but they nearly gave me an ulcer, so I stopped.

"Then I tried kava tincture. I found the effects instantaneous, short-acting, and with no hangover. My mood shifted from 'pam-anxiety' to 'relaxation-uplifting.' I felt great! I like the fact that I can 'titrate' the effect because of its fast onset. I can add a few more drops under the tongue if the first few are not enough. Other times, I just mix it with water. The effect is slightly delayed but the same. I can take it during the day as well. It stops the pain but, unlike the benzodiazepines, I'm still able to concentrate and work."

The other medication Jerry was referring to was a non-steroidal anti-inflammatory (NSAID), such as Advil or Motrin, often prescribed for this type of pain. These can cause irritation of the stomach lining and ulcers.

Kava is an over-the-counter sleeping compound that is also a daytime analgesic, a muscle relaxant, and a mood enhancer, all-in-one, and with no side effects. It saddens me to think of all the people who could benefit from a simple, inexpensive, natural remedy, and instead are given ineffective drugs with side effects.

Since insomnia increases with age, many elderly patients are given benzodiazepines, often with disastrous results. Since their livers are less efficient due to age and they are also using other prescription drugs, elderly people are often taking more medication than their bodies can handle. Forgetfulness is an additional problem, and they may take their dose twice! They tend to suffer from falls, which result in head injuries or hip fractures. Both are dangerous, one adding to an already confused mind, the other often leading to complications that can be fatal.

As we'll discuss in Chapter 9, kava has proved effective in treating insomnia, especially when combined with other herbs, such as valerian.

# Menopause

Numerous clinicians, myself included, have found kava to be useful in treating the physical and psychological symptoms that often accompany menopause: anxiety, irritability, depression, insomnia, and hot flashes. Many women also report relief from premenstrual syndrome (PMS) and menstrual cramps. The Pacific Islanders also used kava for these purposes, owing to its muscle-relaxing properties and sleep stabilizing effects.

A good example is my patient Deanna, a 47-year-old secretary and mother of two adult children, ages 22 and 25, who were no longer living at home.

### Kava's Use for Menopausal Symptoms

Deanna and her husband, Paul, had finally reached the point in their lives where they could have some time to themselves. But Deanna found herself becoming increasingly irritable, moody, and hypercritical. Much to her dismay (and everyone else's), Deanna began losing her temper both at home and at work. She also suffered from insomnia and fatigue, and just didn't feel like herself anymore. Unaware that she was actually approaching menopause, Deanna was baffled as to the cause. I explained to her what was going on. The hormonal shifts of "perimenopause" (impending menopause) will often occur before any changes in menstrual patterns. (For more details, see Ann Louise Gittleman's book *Before the Change*.) To Deanna, that in itself was some relief: "I'm not losing my mind after all."

She still needed help to relieve the stress and muscle tension; elevate her moods; and get some solid, deep sleep. I prescribed a daily dose of kava: 70 mg of kavalactones per dose, two to three doses daily, with a third dose (or even two more) at bedtime. I also prescribed a combination of other herbs: valerian, hops, vitex, schizandra, and dong quai. The combination worked wonders: Deanna's symptoms began to ease, and she and Paul were able to start enjoying their new-found freedom. Who knows what they're doing now during those long evenings together!

———————

Research bears out these results. In two placebo-controlled, double-blind studies of a total of 80 women with menopause, related symptoms, the kava groups had significant reductions in anxiety symptoms, hot flashes, and other menopausal symptoms. They also had improvements in sleep, mood, and a subjective sense of well-being. The placebo groups showed no significant changes.[13, 14]

## Kava and Kids

Though kava drinking in the Pacific was an activity typically restricted to adult males, young boys or girls were selected to chew the roots to prepare it for drinking. Additionally, drinking a beverage of the "nene" variety was used to calm "nervous children." Here in the West, society strongly opposes children's involvement with drugs or alcohol. At the same time, apparently oblivious to the inconsistency, powerful drugs such as Ritalin and Prozac are prescribed in huge numbers to treat a near epidemic of childhood hyperactivity, Attention Deficit Disorder, and other behavioral and emotional problems.

Might kava provide a safe, natural alternative? Few, if any, studies have been done on the effectiveness of kava with children, but the herb's mildness and demonstrated calming effects would seem to make it a good fit. I believe one should exercise caution in giving any psychoactive substance to a child. However, when one looks at the above-mentioned psychotropic drugs, which are routinely prescribed to youngsters, kava appears to be quite benign in comparison. One of my patients Jerry (the earlier insomnia case), reports using kava with his children to help them transition at bedtime, and says it works wonders.

Matt and Valerie, ages four and six, are good kids, bright and active, with a lot of energy. As bedtime approaches, they occasionally become a bit *too* active and difficult—cranky, whiny, argumentative, and unwilling to go to bed peacefully. Jerry discovered that a few drops of kava, combined with warm milk and a story, makes for a relatively painless bedtime. The children calm down and become their natural angelic selves. After a quiet story, they drift off into the deep, restful sleep for which kava is famous.

## Beyond Relaxation: Other Medical Uses

Aside from its considerable potential to alleviate stress, kava's other properties make it a promising natural remedy for a variety of other ailments, as we will see in Table 8.1 on page 108. Over the centuries in different cultures, kava has been used as a diuretic, a diaphoretic (to induce sweating during colds and fevers), as a cure for rheumatism and asthma, and as a cure for worms. It has also been used to relieve headaches, promote sleep and relieve fatigue, and to treat skin diseases such as fungal infections and leprosy. It has long been considered safe enough to give to children. Kava's first popularity in Europe was in Germany during the 1890s, when patent remedies were sold as urinary tract anti-septics and diuretics.

Here in the West, we have not begun to extensively explore most of these uses, but I can report on one case. My patient Doreen noticed that when she used kava for sleep, her asthma symptoms improved. She now successfully uses a spray or two of kava when she begins to wheeze.

## Chronic Fatigue Syndrome

Many practitioners of natural medicine, myself included, find kava quite effective against the mysterious and frustrating condition called chronic fatigue syndrome (CFS). Combined with rcishi mushroom, kava is excellent for relieving the symptoms of CFS and fibromyalgia, a form of muscle and connective tissue tenderness that often accompanies this syndrome. Besides the muscle-relaxing effect, kava appears to work directly on the limbic system, the emotional center of the human brain. This promotes a sense of well-being, relieving the depression that so often accompanies this disorder.

## Local Anesthesia

Kava's numbing properties have interested some scientists in the herb's potential as an anesthetic. In 1939, researcher A. G. Van Veen determined that the kavalactone kavain was as effective and long-lasting as cocaine in inducing local anesthesia. Cocaine is the source of a number of topical and injectable anesthetics, including lidocaine, marcaine, and novocaine. However, the potential of high doses to cause

## Table 8.1. Kava in Traditional Medicine

The following chart describes some of the traditional medicinal uses of kava throughout the islands. These are of ethno-medical interest only, and not meant to be suggested home remedies.

| Condition | Treatment |
|---|---|
| Inflammation of urogenital system | Drinking macerated stump and young kava shoots |
| Gonorrhea and chronic cystitis | Drinking prepared kava |
| Menstrual problems | Drinking prepared kava |
| Difficulties urinating | Drinking macerated stump |
| Rheumatism | Drinking macerated stump |
| Weight gain | Drinking macerated stump |
| Irritation of respiratory tract | Drinking macerated stump |
| Asthma | Drinking macerated stump |
| Female puberty syndromes, weakness | Drinking masticated kava |
| Migraine related to women's sicknesses | Drinking masticated kava |
| To prevent infection | Drinking masticated kava |
| Pulmonary pains | Drinking masticated kava |
| Vaginal prolapsus | Application of macerated kava |

paralysis in peripheral nerves made one researcher wary of kavain's suitability for the role. But in lower doses, kava applied topically to the skin appears to be safe and effective for minor irritations.[15]

"Anyone who's chewed or drank kava knows of its powerful topical anesthetic properties," says kava importer Gary Friedman. "I'm surprised more products haven't been developed to take advantage of that. In the Pacific Islands, they

**Table 8.1. Kava in Traditional Medicine**

| Condition | Treatment |
|---|---|
| To provoke abortion | Kava leaves in vagina |
| Headaches | Masticated root tissues, eaten or drunk as an infusion |
| General weakness | Drinking of masticated, macerated kava diluted with water and boiled |
| Chills and sleeping problems | Drinking of masticated, macerated kava diluted with water and boiled |
| Chills | Drinking macerated kava; fumigation with lcavcs |
| General treatment of disease | Fumigation with leaves |
| Gastrointestinal upset | Drinking macerated stump mixed with other medicinal plants |
| Tuberculosis | Drinking juice extracted from stump |
| Leprosy | External application of masticated stump |
| Skin diseases | Application of poultice of masticated stump[16] |

have kava chewing gum and toothpastes for people with sensitive gums. And in Aruba, they're experimenting with using a kava-based lotion for insect bites." We have recently seen an herbal sore throat spray on the market, which touts that it is effective "for temporary relief of pain and irritation." It "contains kava rather than phenol, a known carcinogen used in other over-the-counter throat sprays". This appears to be a less toxic approach along with the other benefits of kava.

## Antifungal

---

Although, as was noted above, kava has been used traditionally as an antibacterial, *in vitro* (test tube) studies failed to establish significant antibacterial activity.[17] On the other hand, some of the kavalactones have shown antifungal properties against a wide array of pathogenic fungi.[18] It is speculated that the kavalactones may undergo chemical changes within the body that would not show up in in vitro studies, but might explain its success with urinary tract infections[19, 20]

## Bladder Infections

---

"Hardly anyone is using kava to treat bladder infections, even though it's tremendously effective," says Terry Willard. "Kava is a known antifungal, and just as kava numbs the mouth, it also anesthetizes the bladder and urinary tract while relaxing the pelvic area, all of which makes it a good symptomatic treatment for bladder infections, especially in women." Kava's muscle-relaxing properties help calm the spasms that often accompany urinary tract infections that empty the bladder.

   In the next chapter, we discuss how kava affects sleep and insomnia, and the causes and treatments for both.

## CHAPTER 9

# Sleep and Insomnia

A s we say throughout this book, life is complex, and its highest goal seems to be achieving and sustaining dynamic balance in all its systems—physical, mental, emotional, and social. Sleep is an essential part of that balance. Nearly all animals and even some plants undergo some form of sleep on a regular basis. In sleep, creatures rest, repair, and rejuvenate themselves. Our body is governed by dozens of interrelated cycles of internal clocks. These are the internal rhythms that control and coordinate hormone production, hunger, moods, body temperature, and energy level. Many of these are related to our patterns of sleeping and waking.

As with our body's apparent overstimulation of the stress response, our prehistoric genetic blueprint for sleep has not evolved quickly enough to keep pace with our emerging twenty-four-hour-a-day lives. According to sleep experts, if you want to be fully alert, in a good mood, mentally sharp, creative, and energetic all day, you might need to spend at least one-third of your life sleeping; that means eight hours a night.

"People have no idea how important sleep is to their lives," says Thomas Roth, Ph.D., health and scientific advisor of the National Sleep Foundation and director of the Sleep Disorders Research Center at Henry Ford Hospital in Detroit. "Good health demands good sleep. Conversely, lack of sleep and sleep problems have serious, often life-threatening consequences."[1]

Today, more than one in three people boast of sleeping six hours or less. They consider themselves tough, motivated, and disciplined. Yet even minimal sleep loss can have profound effects on all aspects of our lives. We're less alert and attentive, more irritable and moody, and our relationships suffer. As our concentration and judgment diminish and our ability to perform even simple tasks declines, our true productivity shrinks. At the same time, accident rates increase, as do health problems, particularly those in our gastrointestinal, cardiovascular, and immune systems.

When we lose sleep or our sleep is of poor quality, we also put ourselves and those around us at high risk for accidents. Perhaps nothing brings this home more clearly than the following finding by Stanley Coren, professor of psychology at the University of British Columbia. Coren found that there is a 7% increase in accidental deaths in the four days after we lose one hour of sleep following the spring shift to daylight saving time, compared to the week before and the week after. The pattern is reversed in the fall, when we gain an hour's sleep for one night.[2]

Drowsy drivers cause at least 100,000 highway accidents and 1,500 deaths in the U.S. each year.[3] According to the National Highway Traffic Safety Administration, more than half of all adults have driven while drowsy in the past year, with 31% acknowledging that they had actually fallen asleep behind the wheel.[4]

Thomas Edison's proudest invention—electric lighting—ruined people's sleep habits. Before that invention, most people slept an average of ten hours a night. In the 1950s and 1960s, the average dropped to eight, and it now hovers around seven and continues to fall. The trend is similar throughout the world.[5, 6]

## A "Doing" Society

Nike knows as a society we like to "just do it." As a culture, we don't respect or value being, dreaming, or sleeping. As a result, not only do we not spend enough time on it—time is money, after all—but we don't know enough about it. There is a serious need for more research into sleep, its effects, and how best to promote and support it. However, what we do know is cause for concern, as indicated in the sidebar "Sobering Statistics About American Sleep Habits," on page 114.

In the past 25 years, we've added 158 hours to our annual work and commuting time—a full month of working hours.[7] According to William C. Dement, M.D., Ph.D., the director of the Sleep Disorders Clinic and Laboratory at the Stanford University School of Medicine, working mothers with young children have added 241 hours to their work and commuting schedules since 1969. Dement passionately believes ". . . Americans need to wake up to the crucial importance of sleep in their lives."[8]

Natural immune system modulators, such as interleukin and tumor necrosis factor, increase during slow-wave sleep.[9] Studies by Dr. Michael Irwin and colleagues at the University of California San Diego and San Diego Veterans Affairs Medical Center suggest that even a modest loss of sleep reduces the body's immune response. Twenty-three healthy men, aged 22–64, spent four nights in a sleep lab. They were allowed to sleep normally the first two nights, but

### Sobering Statistics About American Sleep Habits

- The amount of Americans that suffer sleeplessness at some point in their lives—many chronically—is 50%.

- Seven hours per weekday night is the average amount of sleep for men and women in the United States—in suburban, urban, and rural areas.

- The amount of adults that now report daytime drowsiness as a problem is 56%.

- The amount of people who report being so sleepy during the day that it interferes with daily activities is 37%; the figure is 52% among shift workers.

- Among those who report daytime sleepiness, 30% report a drop in job performance and 50% report a drop in performance of family duties.

- The amount of American adults that report a sleep-related problem is 67% (a 33% increase in five years).

the third night they were kept awake from 3:00 to 7:00 A.M. The following morning, for 18 of the men, the activity of the immune cells that fight off viral infections fell significantly. When the men were allowed to sleep through the next night uninterrupted, the level of immune cells returned to normal. This indicates that sleep deprivation—even one-half night of lost sleep—decreases the body's ability to ward off infection.[10]

The National Sleep Foundation points to our escalating pace of life, work pressures, and aging as the primary reasons many medical specialists now believe sleep disorders to be the number one health problem in America.[11, 12]

- The amount who suffer from insomnia is 43%.

- Thirty million suffer from sleep apnea (temporary cessation of breathing), a potentially life-threatening disorder.

- The amount who report symptoms consistent with restless leg syndrome is 15%.[13]

- The amount of money spent on direct medical costs of sleep disorders and sleep deprivation in 1990 was $15.9 billion.

- The amount of money spent on indirect costs, such as productivity and accidents, in 1990 was $150 billion.[14]

- The amount of people with sleep disorders that go undiagnosed and untreated is 95%.[15]

- The amount of money lost per year in productivity, accidents, and health-related costs as a result of workers' inability to adjust to late night work schedules is $70 billion.[16]

# Stages of Sleep

To accomplish its critical role of rejuvenation, sleep is a dynamic process with a complex "architecture" all its own. Though the overall level of neural activity drops by only 10%, the brain's receptivity to outside stimuli is greatly restricted through a sharp decline in the activity of the reticular activating system (RAS) within the brain stem. We survive, however, because major stimuli, such as an earthquake or a car alarm, gets through to the brain. Living in Los Angeles, one can count on being rudely awakened by either of these.

Sleep labs monitor sleep patterns through the use of electrodes attached to specific locations on a subject's face and scalp. The electroencephalograph (EEG) monitors brain wave activity, the electro-oculogram (EOG), monitors eye movements, and the electromyogram (EMG) records electrical changes in muscles. Physiological changes are recorded on graph paper in a series of lines that resemble the jagged outlines of a mountain range.

When a subject is awake and alert, the EEG records the firing of millions of individual nerve cells in a series of fast and choppy squiggles called *alpha* and *beta* waves. Beta waves dominate during periods of mental arousal and tension, and alpha waves dominate when one is quietly relaxed. *Delta,* or *theta,* waves are the larger, slower EEG tracings recorded during non-REM (rapid eye movement) sleep.

There are two stages of relaxation before sleep, and four more stages before the period of rapid eye movements or REMs begin. Sleep is preceded by what is termed *sleep latency.* Your eyes are closed, and your muscles are deeply relaxed, as you drowsily drift toward Stage 1, where you lose consciousness. This light sleep lasts several minutes, and your brain waves are irregular and rapid.

In Stage 2, brain waves become larger and slower, with brief bursts of electrical activity called *sleep spindles.* Your blood pressure and heart rate decrease, as you become increasingly detached from your surroundings. This intermediate stage lasts about half an hour.

Then you move into deep non-REM sleep Stages 3 and 4, in which the brain produces large, slow waves. Body temperature drops, and blood pressure and heart rate continue to decrease, as you become more difficult to awaken. Often called "delta" or slow-wave sleep, this is physically restorative sleep, as cells start to repair and rejuvenate. These stages may be decreased or absent in the elderly, who awaken more frequently during the night.

After an hour or so, you shift into a highly active stage characterized by accelerated dreaming and rapid eye movements, hence the name REM sleep. Though we may dream in all stages of sleep, dreams occur most frequently in REM sleep and are usually more vivid and emotional than during other stages. This stage is also called "paradoxical sleep" because while your brain waves are suddenly almost the same as if you were awake, the brain sends out signals that relax the large muscle groups in the body so thoroughly that they are literally paralyzed. This has survival value, in that it stops people from physically acting out their dreams.

It is primarily during REM that our bodies and minds are refreshed and rejuvenated. Newborns spend almost 50% of their sleep time in REM; by three months, REM is only 30%. At six months, it's down to 20%.[17] In rapidly growing young adults, it rises again to 25%. For most adults, REM sleep occurs every 90 minutes throughout the night. The first REM period is brief, lasting around five minutes. As each REM period ends, you ascend back into non-REM sleep, and then cycle between them for the rest of the night. As the night progresses, REM periods become longer, up to 30–45 minutes, and REM becomes a dominant part of the sleep cycle.

Science is still debating the precise role of each sleep stage. Delta wave sleep seems to allow the body to recover, while REM sleep and dreams work to restore the brain, including storing, organizing, updating, and discarding information. Without enough REM sleep, it becomes harder to focus on day-to-day activities. Also, it is believed that during the dreaming of the REM phase, the subconscious mind analyzes the day's events and processes feelings, also essential for mental health.

## Insomnia

Insomnia affects 20% to 43% of American adults at some point in their lives. Insomnia most commonly consists of

## Table 9.1 Causes and Treatments for Insomnia

| Causes of Insomnia | Possible Treatments |
| --- | --- |
| Stress, depression, anxiety | Psychotherapy and/or medication |
| Irregular sleep schedule | A regular sleep/wake schedule |
| Associating bed with alert activities | Relaxing bedtime schedules |
| Exercising too close to bedtime | Exercising earlier in the day |
| Caffeine | No caffeine |
| Excessive alcohol intake or abuse | No evening alcohol |
| Nicotine | No smoking |

increased sleep latency, or difficulty falling asleep. In fact, 50% of senior citizens have difficulty falling asleep on any given night.[18]

The National Sleep Foundation (NSF) identifies three categories of insomnia: transient, short-term, and chronic. Transient insomnia lasts only a few nights and is usually brought on by particular stress, excitement, or a change in sleep timing or environment. Short-term insomnia recurs for two or three weeks, and can be caused by ongoing stress, as well as medical or psychiatric problems. Anxiety, grief, loneliness, changing jobs, or the loss of a loved one are some of the causes of short-term insomnia. Alleviating the source will usually return sleep to normal, though recurring episodes are common. Chronic insomnia afflicts 15% of adults, 50% of the elderly. It lasts more than a month and sometimes for decades. It can be related to underlying medical, behavioral, or psychiatric problems, such as depression, possibly involving a serotonin imbalance in the brain.

The NSF also suggests six major origins of insomnia: psychiatric problems, psychological problems, preexisting medical issues, poor sleep hygiene, circadian rhythm factors (such as a change in work shifts), or learned insomnia (where insomnia continues after the initial stimulus has been removed).

Insomnia rarely exists in a vacuum, and is often viewed as a symptom of an underlying problem, much like a fever suggests infection. Sufferers generally have other psychiatric disorders that are leading them to feel distress, such as anxiety and depression. Or, they may have more serious underlying physical disturbances including hyperthyroidism, endocrine imbalance, diabetes, hypoglycemia, fibromyalgia, arthritis, cardiac and respiratory problems, sleep apnea, restless leg syndrome, or drug and alcohol abuse. See Table 9.1 on page 118 for a list of various causes and treatments for insomnia.

It is important, therefore, to undertake a full investigation of what could be contributing to insomnia before suggesting or undertaking a specific treatment. Unfortunately, only about half the people suffering from sleep disturbances seek the advice of a health-care professional, and many of these individuals are prescribed sleeping pills, while the underlying disorder causing the insomnia goes untreated.

## Age and Sleep

Although the ability to sleep well may diminish with age, the need for sleep does not. In addition to specific sleep disorders, older people are more likely to suffer medical problems that can interrupt, delay, and/or shorten sleep, as may some of the drugs used to treat these conditions.

The average total sleep time increases slightly after age 65, but so do reports of difficulty falling asleep. One study found that after age 65, 13% of men and 36% of women reported taking more than 30 minutes to fall asleep. Research suggests that physiological changes are partially at fault. The elderly generally secrete lesser amounts of certain chemicals (including melatonin, which is discussed later in this chapter) that regulate the sleep/wake cycle. Changes in the body temperature cycle that can affect sleep also occur with age.

Lifestyle changes and behavioral practices may also play a part. Daytime naps may make us less tired at bedtime. Poor sleep habits may have become entrenched. For example, we may associate our beds with television or reading, rather than sleeping. The need to use the bathroom more frequently may make nighttime risings necessary. Some researchers theorize that daytime inactivity (lack of exercise) and decreased mental stimulation may also lead to the "aging" of sleep.

Sometimes, age-related changes mask underlying sleep disorders. For example, sleep apnea, a breathing disorder, is more common in the middle and elder years. The repeated awakenings caused by a literal lack of breath lead to daytime sleepiness.

## Pharmaceutical Medications

According to the National Sleep Foundation, in the treatment of transient and short-term insomnia "sleeping pills have a role" but "once the source of the stress or disruption is dealt with or improved sleep hygiene shows positive effects, medications are discontinued, usually within two weeks." In chronic insomnia, "sleeping pills have a limited role and are not intended for long-term use." Most medical authorities recommend that benzodiazepine use be limited to four weeks.[19]

Despite the fact that drug therapy is recommended only as temporary sleep support, approximately 7% of the population take medication regularly, 13% use prescription sedatives, and 87% use over-the-counter (OTC) products. The OTC products include depressants and antihistamines that slow brain activity and cause drowsiness. These drugs break down slowly in the body, and produce next-day drowsiness. While they may help with occasional or mild insomnia, they don't work with continued use, for which they were never intended. They should be used only under doctor's supervision by those with glaucoma, peptic ulcer, seizure disorder, or prostate enlargement.

# Benzodiazepines

It is estimated that American doctors write 25 million prescriptions a year for sedative-hypnotic drugs like Valium. Besides anxiety, insomnia is the most common reason that people take benzodiazepines. There is almost unanimous agreement that these drugs effectively induce sleep, reduce latency, and increase total sleep time for the first several nights.

Side effects include morning sleepiness, rebound insomnia, and disruption in thinking. While they may induce a good night's sleep, with many of the benzodiazepines, their effects last several days. With significant amounts still in their systems, users are "hung over" the next day, and their level of alertness is impaired.

An American Psychiatric Association Task Force reported the risk of increases in traffic accidents after patients are given a prescription for benzodiazepines. Those who filled three prescriptions in a six-month period had an even higher risk.[20] In a study of 300,000 people, the risk of traffic accidents was significantly greater for users than for those in the control group. While the risk was highest during the week after the prescription was filled, it remained higher even four weeks later.[21] This is not to say that the prescriptions caused the accidents; after all, these people were likely troubled by anxiety or insomnia before they sought help.

# Benzodiazepines and the Elderly

Since insomnia increases with age, many elderly patients are given benzodiazepines, often with disastrous results. Those over 65 comprise about 15% of the population, yet they consume up to 45% of sleep medications, and 40% of the nation's benzodiazepines.

The negative effects are worse for them, and there is far too little awareness of this phenomenon. A particularly tragic effect of the benzodiazepines is an increase in accidents due to a loss of muscle coordination, which appears to strike the aged more than younger patients.[22]

## Rose, Esther, and Overuse of Benzodiazepines

### *Background*

Esther, the 77-year-old mother of one of my patients, came in to see me. Ever since her husband Ralph died six years earlier, she'd grown very close to her best friend, Rose. Rose was a couple of years younger, but according to Esther, "you wouldn't know it to see her these days." Since both their husbands had died within a few months of each other, they'd become nearly inseparable. But a few months ago, according to Esther, "Rose's sleeping problems got worse and worse. She wasn't remembering as well, and she was complaining more. She wasn't having as much fun, and so she wasn't as much fun to be with.

"Then her doctor gave her some pills to help her sleep. He said it would also help her nerves. She said she slept better, but she also seemed somewhat confused and forgetful. Then she fell and broke her hip, and her kids put her in a rest home. They said it was just until she got on her feet again. But she's not getting better. I miss her. Since her fall, we don't see each other nearly as much. And I'm starting to have trouble sleeping. I don't want to take what she's taking. What should I do?"

*Treatment*

Esther's insomnia wasn't severe yet. It hadn't begun to feed on itself, where lack of sleep makes it harder to sleep. But she had taken her friend's problems and absence very hard, and she was scared—of loss, of things going downhill, and of dying. She confessed to me that her kids had always called her "a cockeyed optimist," but she was having trouble lately living up to the name.

Besides just listening to her, which she sorely needed, I recommended some supplements and kava, once or twice during the day for her anxiety, and a kava sleep combination before bed for sleep (see Chapter 12). The treatment worked. She was able to relax and to feel a bit more like herself, and she slept well.

A few weeks later, Esther was much better, and she asked if I would talk to Rose about kava. I saw Rose and gradually shifted her off the benzodiazepines and on to an herbal program similar to Esther's. Rose was able to move back home, and both she and Esther come to see me together on occasion for maintenance. They joke about taking a cruise to the South Seas and drinking kava from coconut shells.

---

For seniors, physical exercise and engagement with others are crucial to physical and mental health. A hip fracture or similar debilitating accident can ultimately be a death sentence—in terms of the likelihood of immobilization leading to deterioration of health, and the onset of illnesses, such as pneumonia, more serious at that age.

## Benzodiazepines: Tolerance and Addiction

At any age, benzodiazepines quickly produce a tolerance, so that one has to increase dosage to achieve results. Worst of

## Statistics on the Elderly and Benzodiazepines

- In a study of 16,000 people over age 65, the risk of traffic accidents was significantly greater for those taking benzodiazepines.[23]

- In the United States, falls are a leading cause of accidental death in people over age 65.[24, 25]

- Falls contribute to 40% of nursing home admissions.

- Five percent of falls result in hip fractures and other injuries that require hospitalization or immobilization for an extended period.[26]

- The elderly have both a higher risk of falling and a higher rate of hip fractures when taking benzodiazepines.[27]

- In one study involving 6,000 patients, those taking flurezepam, diazepam, or chlordiazepoxide had a risk of hip fracture 1.8 times greater than those not taking the drug.[28]

- In a study of 100 hospital patients age 70 and over who had fallen, and 100 controls (also over age 70) who had not fallen, there was a higher rate of falls associated with benzodiazepine use.[29]

all, 15% to 30% of long-term users become addicted. Most research has shown that their beneficial effects for sleep last only a few weeks, yet many patients feel unable to sleep without them after months or even years of use.[30]

A critical study in 1988 examined the difference between what is reported in the scientific literature and the subjective experiences of people who take benzodiazepines. Forty subjects with chronic insomnia, who had been on benzodiazepines for six months or more and felt unable to stop the drug even though they wanted to, were compared with 36 people with chronic insomnia who did not take sleeping aids.

After initial evaluations comparing the two groups, patients who had been prescribed benzodiazepines stopped taking them and further comparison was made. Evaluation of the sleep of these groups of patients was done with polysomnographic recordings (EEG, EOG, EMG) throughout the entire night, as well as subjective evaluation of sleep by all the patients.

Sleep duration was the same in both groups. REM sleep, however, was significantly reduced in people who took benzodiazepines. When people stopped taking their medication, sleep duration increased in 21 patients and decreased in 19 patients, but most significantly, there was a dramatic increase of REM sleep in all 40 of the patients.[31]

# How Important Is REM?

Long, deep sleep ending with a lot of REM sleep helps consolidate learning, while failure to get proper sleep can wipe it out. Dreams during REM may be nonsensical for the same reason that housecleaning tends to make things messier before it makes them cleaner.

- Positron emission tomography (PET) scans of the brain show metabolic activity associated with learning to be significantly higher during REM sleep than during non-REM sleep or wakefulness

- Cerebral glucose metabolism seems to indicate that REM sleep promotes memory[32]

- REM activity is more intense following periods of intensive learning[33]

- Performance studies show dramatic improvement in memory retention after REM sleep, compared to non-REM sleep or equivalent time awake

- On the other hand, subjects deprived of REM sleep find it difficult to retain recently learned material[34]

- Adequate REM sleep seem to be particularly important for peak daytime performance that calls for memory retention and recall[35]

Neurotransmitters such as norepinephrine and serotonin are considered crucial for new learning and retention. During REM sleep, the brain's neurotransmitter supply is replenished. By inhibiting neurotransmitter restoration, the lack of quality sleep interferes with the ability to learn and remember.[36] Just think of all the prescriptions written for neurotransmitter-enhancing antidepressants, when the underlying problem is actually sleep deprivation. As we have seen, the very drugs given to treat these symptoms prolong and exacerbate them.

Adequate REM is vital for memory storage, retention, organization, reorganization, and new learning. A good analogy is that REM sleep is like running a cleanup program on your computer. During the day we generate a lot of open and disconnected circuits, and probably end up with plenty of fragmented and corrupted files. Unless we run our nightly cleanup, the next day our human computer is likely to run slower and less efficiently, to say nothing of the occasional system errors and total crashes we're likely to face.

A recent study at Rush-Presbyterian-St. Luke's Medical Center in Chicago, Illinois, revealed that increased REM sleep time contributes significantly toward reducing negative mood overnight. Researchers measured overnight mood and depression change in 30 men and 30 women using mood and depression scales combined with sleep and dream content measurements collected over two nights in a sleep lab to observe these results.[37]

All of this illustrates why the effects of REM deficiency, sleep deprivation, and fatigue often develop a self-perpetuating cycle:

- Decreased sleep reduces REM
- Reduced REM prevents rejuvenation
- Unrejuvenated, we are more susceptible to stress
- Feeling stressed decreases sleep

## Sleep and Wake Refreshed with Kava

Having created a social epidemic of sleep deprivation, we need now to turn away from drugs that basically knock us unconscious, then rob us of our precious restorative REM sleep. In addition to its ability to promote calm and well-being, kava may provide an effective natural treatment for insomnia. In an appropriately increased dosage, kava seems to work with the body to bring on deep restful sleep without interfering with sleep's natural cycles.

"Kava . . . does not cloud thought processes before inducing the desire to sleep," according to Vincent Lebot.[38] More specifically, in the islands, "half a coconut shell of kava, containing 1 to 1.5 g of kavalactone resin, induces a deep sleep within 30 minutes—an effect comparable to many conventional drugs. But importantly, the next sleep within 30 minutes an effect comparable to many conventional drugs. But importantly, the next day the user reports no after-effects such as drowsiness or low energy levels."[39]

## Sleeping Pills Linked to Early Mortality

In May 1998, researchers at the University of California at San Diego reported that people who regularly take prescrip-

## A Study of Kava and Sleep

The effect of kava on sleep was demonstrated in a 1991 German study by Emser and Bartylla, in which 12 subjects in their 20s and 30s were divided into two groups, each receiving either 50 mg or 100 mg of standardized kava extract three times a day. For four days and nights, responses were recorded using EEG, EMG, and EEG polygraphic devices. Much like prescription sedatives, kava enhanced EEG sleep spindle density by 20% in 11 out of 12 subjects, regardless of dosage. The time it took to fall asleep was reduced, and deep and slow-wave sleep increased without changes in the REM phase. The higher kava dose produced tendencies to decrease Stage 1 sleep as well as the duration of the wake phase. Subjects reported no rebound in REM sleep when they stopped taking kava. The study concluded that kava supports the natural course of sleep cycles, unlike conventional sedative drugs, which often suppress deep and REM sleep.[40]

Though this study seems to corroborate traditional and clinical experience, it is just one study. With the enormous call for safe and effective sleep aids, there is a need for more research on kava and sleep. Having said that, let us point to one possible explanation for kava's positive properties: Kava has been shown to act on the brain's prime emotion center, the almond-shaped amygdala, which is also known to receive strong stimulation from the brainstem during REM sleep. The exact significance of this remains to be seen.

tion sleeping pills run a greater risk of dying early than those who do not. Even occasional use of the pills, including flurazepam (Dalmane), temazepam (Restoril), and triazolam (Halcion), was associated with an elevation of risk.

According to Dr. Daniel Kripke, who headed the study, "Overall, the hazard associated with taking sleeping pills at least 30 times a month was similar to the hazard of smoking one to two packs of cigarettes per day." Kripke pointed out that today's most popular sleeping pill, zolpidem (Ambien), was not in use at the time of the study, and also cautioned that the study did not show that the pills caused the deaths.[41] We acknowledge that those who take 30 sleeping pills a month may have various other possible causes of early death.

# Other Sleep Aids

## *Melatonin*

The hormone melatonin is instrumental in establishing our daily rhythms. As we age, our melatonin levels decrease, with the steepest decline occurring after 50. Melatonin supplements may play a role in restoring internal sleeping and waking rhythms, as it works on an underlying physiological cause of sleep disorder. In an Israeli study at the Technion Medical School in Haifa, men and women between the ages of 68 to 80, had their time to fall asleep cut by more than half (from 40 minutes to 15 minutes), with the use of melatonin. They also reported their sleep was more refreshing.

Walter Pierpaoli and William Riegelson, M.D., in their book *The Melatonin Miracle* recommend 1 to 5 mg at bedtime.[42] They suggest you begin with 1 mg the first night, and if it works, continue with that dose. If it doesn't work, increase by 1 mg each night, but only up to a 5 mg maximum. If you wake groggy, they suggest you cut back. Your internal clock should be reset after about two weeks, at which point they recommend you discontinue melatonin.

In my practice, I will suggest melatonin in the same manner for short-term, low-dose use. While its popularity has increased due to its possible antiaging effects, it is still a hormone that needs to be appropriately prescribed and monitored.

### Serotonin and St. John's Wort

Sleep disorders are sometimes linked with lowered brain levels of the neurotransmitter serotonin. Normally before sleep, serotonin levels build up, and at a certain point, the sleep response begins. Melatonin, a metabolite of serotonin, is also involved. Where inadequate levels of serotonin are the problem, antidepressant drugs known as SSRIs, which selectively inhibit serotonin reuptake, can promote sleep. However, these pharmaceuticals have serious side effects, and should be avoided when safer natural treatment is effective. St. John's wort, used in depression and anxiety, likely has a serotonin- and a melatonin-enhancing effect, helping to regulate sleep naturally. Many of my patients notice that their sleep improves markedly after a few weeks on the herb (see Chapter 12). L-tryptophan and 5-hydroxy-tryptophan provide additional alternatives. L-tryptophan is available only by prescription from compounding pharmacies (see Appendix B). Its sale was severely restricted after a contaminated batch in 1989 caused serious negative reactions. 5-HTP, a metabolite of tryptophan, is readily available as a supplement (see Chapter 13).

### Other Sleep-Promoting Herbs

Other sleep-promoting herbs include valerian, California poppy, skullcap, hops, passion flower, and reishi mushroom (see Chapter 12).

## Sleep Promoting Behavior Changes

Our ability to sleep is greatly influenced by simple behavioral habits, patterns, and cues. This is good news. Paying attention and taking responsibility for developing healthy "sleep hygiene" has been shown to result in permanent improvement in people's ability to fall and stay asleep and feel more satisfied with their sleep.[43, 44] There are instructive books on the subject, and although they don't yet provide enough information about herbal treatments, the National Sleep Foundation provides valuable resources.

## A Sleep Log Can Be Effective

Keeping a sleep log for a few weeks may be helpful in identifying behaviors that are contributing to your sleep problem. Record when you wake up, go to sleep, drink caffeinated beverages, exercise, eat, and any other suspected sleep-stealers. Simple changes in daily routine may be surprisingly effective in improving sleep quality.

- Avoid caffeinated beverages. Even if taken early in the day, they can disrupt sleep

- Avoid alcohol and nicotine for at least two hours before bedtime (see Chapter 15).

- Exercise regularly, but not too close to bedtime

- Get up at the same time every day regardless of when you went to sleep

In the next chapters, beginning with Chapter 10, we will provide practical information regarding how to use kava to reap the benefits of this peaceful herb.

## CHAPTER 10

# How to Take Kava

A first-time kava user can be overwhelmed walking into a well-stocked supplement store, with its bewildering array of kava products that vary in brand, dosage, and form of administration. In this chapter, you will learn about the essential forms and doses.

## Dosage

While there are more novel delivery systems entering the market daily, kava basically comes in the following forms:

- Tinctures, alcohol-based
- Tablets
- Soft-gel encased paste

- Encapsulated powdered extract

- Sprays

- Powdered extract

# Delivery Systems

If you desire fast absorption, use the liquid forms—sprays, tinctures, and reconstituted extract.

- Tinctures (generally, alcohol tincture): These can be taken straight from the dropper bottle, but be fore-warned: The combination of kava and alcohol has a very strong taste! It also numbs the inside of your mouth, as mentioned in Chapter 1. You can dilute it in warm water, and let the alcohol evaporate before drinking. If the taste is still too overpowering (it's a developed taste), you can add it to juice. Alcohol is also an excellent way to keep kava's active ingredients both well-preserved and soluble, since they don't dissolve well in plain water. For those with alcohol intolerance, there are glycerin-based formulas, where the alcohol used in the extraction process has been removed by evaporation.

- Oral sprays are appearing more regularly in the herbal marketplace. They are quickly absorbed through the mucous membrane for rapid onset. For this same reason, they are also shorter acting. These are good for an anxious moment before going onstage, or for taking final exams.

Tablets and capsules provide a convenient dosing unit, both for measure and portability, and they may become more popular based on the taste factor.

- Tablets tend to dissolve more rapidly than gelcaps.

- Gelcaps are slower to break down and be absorbed in the body. This gives a "slow release" effect, making it longer lasting, which can be an advantage. The extract within is also well-protected from breakdown by exposure to air and may keep its potency longer. *Warning:* In addition to the kava extract paste, the gelcaps generally contain an emulsifier such as lecithin, plus soy oil and beeswax. Make sure that you are not allergic to any of these carriers. Rare though this is, I did have one patient who was allergic to bee products, and couldn't tolerate the gelcaps. She did fine, however, on the tincture.

- Hard-gelatin powder-filled capsules or, for those who prefer non-animal based products, vegetable-based capsules are a common form. These are not simply powdered kava root, but solvent-extracted material, dried, sprayed on a base, and encapsulated.

Traditional drinks aside, this is the order of speed of delivery of commercial products:

- Sprays (provide the most immediate effects, followed by tinctures)

- Powdered extracts

- Tablets and hard-gelatin capsules

- Soft gel capsules

## Dosage Information

To begin with, look for extract that is standardized, meaning that there is a consistent amount of the active ingredients. Standardization also permits researchers to define the composition and strength of a product, both for replication of studies and for practical, clinical purposes.

Most kava researchers have used a dosing unit of 100 mg of 70% kavalactones, which yields 70 mg of kavalactones. This high concentration has not been available commercially, nor is it necessary. In fact, preparations containing 30% kavalactones are generally clinically superior to those of higher concentrations. In the higher concentrations, you are likely to lose the contribution of other, as-yet unidentified constituents.

The important factor is the total content of kavalactone by weight. Most commercial products contain 200 to 250 mg of 30% kavalactones, yielding 60 to 75 mg per capsule or tablet. This is approximately the same amount by weight as 100 mg of the 70% extract, which yields 70 mg. By way of comparison, one shell of drinking kava typically contains 250 mg of lactones, the equivalent of nearly four of these doses, and islanders often polish off four or five shells in a sitting, equaling 1,000 mg.

The recommended clinical dosage for adults, for general anxiety or stress relief:

- Seventy to 210 mg daily, in divided doses. That is, one capsule, tablet, or dose of tincture, at intervals throughout the day, for a total of three per day. The total dose of kavalactones should not exceed 300 mg per day, or four doses of 70 mg each.

- With most tinctures, the dose is 40 drops, three to four times a day.

For sleep:

- Seventy to 210 mg, or up to three doses at once, one hour before bedtime.

- One to two dropperfuls, adjusted as needed. Since the liquid works more quickly, it can be taken closer to bedtime.

These figures are only guidelines, since we all have different tolerances. If you are particularly sensitive to kava's sedating effects, you can start by taking a 70 mg dose in the evening. Based on the result, you can take an additional dose during the day, increasing over the next five to seven days to a daily total of three doses.

The advantage of using herbs like kava, available without a prescription, is that you can take responsibility for your own choice of product (once you are past the confusion), as well as form and schedule of administration, and can monitor your response as you go along. Even without the exact strength listed on the label, as with some tinctures, the best measure is how you feel.

Because of the varying sources of kava, with different cultivars, technical growers, islands, and extraction processes, there is bound to be some variation in the kavalactone proportions among the end-products. In my practice, I've found that some patients respond better to certain brands and delivery systems than to others, so if one isn't working for you, a switch might be indicated.

### Other Ways to Take Kava

Kava is also available in three other forms:

- Instant powdered extract (less available, as of now). As with the capsules above, this is not the powdered root, but a spray-dried water soluble powder used as an instant drink. Unlike a tablet or capsule that hits a local spot in the stomach and dissolves slowly, the liquid is absorbed all at once, which is closer to the effects of the traditional beverage.

- Powdered kava root. This is closest to the traditional form, and requires you to extract the active ingredients yourself. See Appendix C for a description on how this is done. This form is not for your quick morning dose!

- The real thing. Travel to Vanuatu, and go to a *nakamal,* or participate in a formal kava ceremony, as we did (see Chapter 1). This drink will likely be more psychoactive than the ones commercially available in the United States and Europe, for several reasons: It's fresh, and it's more concentrated. Cultivars are selected for their psychoactive effects, and as with fine vineyards, the best stuff is kept at home.

The majority of kava distributors are marketing kava as a calm, relaxing, safe, dietary supplement, and keeping its more exotic South Pacific cultural history in the closet. Some, like herbal manufacturer Andy Levine, think that "it's a shame that kava has to lose its rich cultural history in order to sell to America. In the South Pacific, it's a revered plant experience. Many other cultures haven't rejected these experiences the way America has. We don't know how to deal with them. Our traditional culture is going to McDonald's. . . ."[1]

### Other Products

There is an ever-expanding variety of new kava products available. There are also teas as well as infusions, to be steeped in cold water, or warm water to heighten the potency. Several beverages or elixirs deliver kava in a flavored (obviously!) drink. Some aim for the appeal of an herbal tonic, while others, some even carbonated, go for that of a healthy soft drink. In addition, we have seen or heard reports of sore throat spray, toothpaste, chewing gum, power bars, chips, cookies, bouillion cubes, and even kava-laced sugar. The list is growing all the time. The questions to ask are: What is the source? Who is the manufacturer? Who is the distributor? Do the products contain enough kava to produce a worthwhile effect? Or are some of these simply cases of slick marketing, taking advantage of a new trend? Many may be of good quality and even effective, but: Caveat emptor! Buyer beware.

### When to Take Kava in Relation to Food

The traditional way for maximum effect, and still recommended, is to take the kava with a little food to enhance absorption, and to help those with sensitive stomaches. A full stomach, however, will inhibit absorption.

# How Long to Use Kava?

The Commission E Report (see Chapter 8) recommends a maximum course of treatment of three months, unless under medical supervision.[2] That's fine if you live in Europe, where most kava is by prescription, but harder to do in the United States, where few doctors have even heard of it.

Kava has a good safety record of centuries of traditional use in the islands, and many years of safe clinical use in Europe. The most recent and longest-running research project was for six months of daily usage, with no ill effects. Positive effects increased with time over the first eight weeks, then remained steady. Other studies, on less disturbed patients, showed results at one week, reaching their maximum at four weeks and continuing.

The rationale in Germany for a three-month limit is not fear of toxicity, as much as a general sense that you shouldn't depend on an outside substance on a daily basis. In dealing with anxiety, kava should be regarded as temporary help while finding ways of healing on a deeper level.

In the next chapter, we will look at issues of safety, and possible side effects, abuse, and addiction.

## CHAPTER 11

# Safety and
# Contraindications

A s we know, kava has been an important social, ritual, and medicinal drink in many Pacific Island cultures for centuries, and it's use is extremely well documented by casual observers and scientists (anthropologists, sociologists) alike. Thus, a good case can be made for defining kava as GRAS, the medical term for "generally recognized as safe." According to the Commission E Report (see Chapter 8), when taken as a standardized extract in the medicinal doses typically prescribed for stress and anxiety, kava possesses no known side effects or toxic consequences.

## Safety and the Commission E Report

In Chapter 8, the Commission E Monograph addresses various safety concerns, including contraindications, duration, and interactions with other drugs. Following, we elaborate on these safety issues.

## Contraindications

According to Commission E, "Kava should not be used during pregnancy, nursing, and endogenous depression." These warnings should be followed; however, for clarification, there have been no published reports of any birth defects, nor any adverse effects in infants of nursing mothers taking kava. Also, as noted later in this chapter, there were no fetal abnormalities found in high dose animal studies. In terms of endogenous depression, this is referring to a more severe form of depression, which may become worse with any anti-anxiety or calming substance. Mild depressive symptoms, on the other hand, can actually benefit from kava, as shown in the studies in Chapter 8.

## Duration

According to Commission E, "Kava should not be taken for more than three months without medical advice." This three-month limit refers to continuous use only, not when taken on an "as needed" basis, which can be done without this restriction. (Kava's advantages for these purposes are that it begins to work immediately, and has no withdrawal problems.) We see, from research, that kava is useful for longer-term continuous treatment. For example, the patients in Volz's 1997 study did well over the six-month course, with minimal side effects (fewer than the placebo group).

## Interactions with Other Drugs

According to Commission E, "Potentiation of effectiveness is possible for substances acting on the central nervous system, such as alcohol, barbiturates, and psychopharmacological agents." A common question is "Can I take kava while I'm taking benzodiazepines or other pharmaceutical antianxiety or antidepressant medication?" Unlike St. John's wort, which can be safely combined with medication during transition under medical supervision, the situation with kava is less clear. In Germany, kava and medication are used together during this transition, with no reported problems. However, this is under the supervision of physicians with experience in this use, and who are taking appropriate precautions. Since we have been unable to establish with certainty the safety of taking kava with the pharmaceuticals, we recommend that you follow a prudent path and start taking kava only *after* you have discontinued the pharmaceutical.

It has been reported that kava "potentiates" (i.e., increases) the sedative effects of barbiturates. In studies done with mice, the kavalactone dihydromethysticin had the greatest effect in this regard (see Chapter 7).We may not be able to extrapolate directly to humans, as demonstrated by the conflicting results between rodents and humans in the kava/alcohol studies described later in this chapter. Further investigation, including more human studies, is needed to answer the questions about kava-drug interaction. Since there may be issues here regarding the safety of such studies, we can start by reviewing any existing information on cases where kava has been mixed with medication.

One report of a possible interaction between kava and a benzodiazepine (Xanax), appears in the dramatically entitled letter to the editor: "Coma from the Health Food Store: Interaction Between Kava and Alprazolam [Xanax]." In the article, doctors describe a 54-year-old male who was admitted to the hospital "in a lethargic and disoriented state" (not in a coma, as the headline states). Moreover, despite the mental impairment, his vital signs (pulse, blood pressure, and temperature) were normal. He recovered within several hours. In addition to taking kava for three days prior, along with continuous use of Xanax (alprazolam), he had also been taking cimetidine (Tagamet) and terazosin (Hytrin).[1]

Xanax is a short-acting benzodiazepine, commonly prescribed for anxiety. There is certainly a possibility of potentiation between the Xanax and kava, though we are not certain how strongly kava affects the GABA binding sites, the sites of action of the benzodiazepines. We have already seen how kava potentiates the sedative effects of barbiturates. However, Germany's Dr. Werner Busse, of the Schwabe Pharmaceutical Co. (manufacturers of the kava), was of the opinion that the Xanax itself can cause accumulation and intensify side effects, as could the other medications. He also noted, referring to conventional medical journals in the United States, that "they seem to be eagerly accepting poorly substantiated and documented reports of possible side effects of botanicals, while being rather reluctant in the past to accept reports on the efficacy of botanicals."

Since kava potentiates the sedative effects of barbiturates, then the possibility of drug interactions between kava and most CNS depressants could be expected. It is reasonable, then, to avoid combining kava and benzodiazepines. If you are currently taking pharmaceuticals and wish to stop, consult your physician or find one who will work with you to shift to herbal treatment. Follow a prudent path to transition yourself from any dependence, and start taking kava only after you have discontinued the pharmaceutical.

# Responsible Consumption/Use

Many people who already take medication are self-treating with herbs and not telling their doctors. Doctors and consumers alike need to have better access to accurate information about herbal products, regarding both beneficial and adverse effects and drug-herb interactions. Once they become educated in this field, pharmacists can be an excellent resource for this information. In the meantime, individuals should use great caution in taking any natural product, particularly psychoactive herbs, when taking prescription medications.

## Mixing Kava and Alcohol

Before the arrival of Europeans, alcohol was unknown in the islands of the Pacific Ocean. White settlers started experimenting with combining kava and alcohol shortly after first contact. To our knowledge, there have been two studies on the combination of alcohol and kava, resulting in two different findings.

When mice were given an oral dose of kava followed by an injection of alcohol, the substances greatly increased each other's sedative action.[2] Human testing, however, showed that kava tends to actually counter some of the safety-related adverse effects of mild alcohol consumption.

Why these apparently conflicting results? The answer likely lies in the relative dose of alcohol; the mice received far higher doses than the humans. Regardless, it appears that a social drinker of kava or ethanol could experience increased intoxication by mixing the two, a fact recognized by many Pacific cultures, which place cultural taboos on mixing the two. We'll give the last word on the subject to nineteenth century explorer William Christian, who observed "If a white trader insists on mixing good kava with bad gin, he has simply to face the consequences. Beer, whiskey, and wine are strictly to be avoided as incompatible with the true kava frame of mind."[3]

## Kava and Driving

In a study of 40 healthy subjects, a standardized dose of kava did not impair their ability to drive or to operate machinery.[4]

Despite this positive finding, caution is recommended regarding driving and kava use, since in higher doses and in more sensitive individuals it can have a sedating effect. See also the Commission E warning.

# Reports of Serious Effects

Initial media reports and a press release by the Los Angeles Police Department implicated kava as the "problem" ingredient responsible for the hospitalization of more than 50 young people following a New Year's Eve "rave" concert in 1997. Labels on a product called "fX Rush," which was given free to concert-goers as a marketing promotion, listed kava as the primary ingredient. The victims' symptoms of dizziness, nausea, shortness of breath, and respiratory arrest, however, are certainly not associated with the mild effects of kava. Subsequent analysis of vials of the product confiscated by the police showed that it contained no kava at all and did contain a toxic chemical. We assume the promoters felt "kava kava" was exotic and unknown enough to attract the interest of the partygoers.

This demonstrates the need for clear and accurate public information regarding emerging herbal products. Also, it is important to be aware of unscrupulous promoters who will make false claims for so-called mind-altering products. Some may even add kava to other products to produce dangerous compounds.

In light of the above story, let us offer a note of caution that holds true with regard to all substances. It is critically important to know to the best of your ability precisely what you are taking, what its effects are, and any potentially dangerous interactions with other substances. In addition, you should know the source of the products you are consuming and be confident that they have not been tampered with.

# No Evidence of Lethal Effects

No one is known to have ever died of kava overdose, compared to thousands of deaths by drug overdose—some accidental and others suicides. Additionally, there are many deaths in accidents caused while driving under the influence of benzodiazepines.

Animal studies give kava a wide margin of safety, with the "lethal dose 50," or LD 50—the amount required to kill half the mice—about 1,000 mg/kg.[5] In studies where dogs and rats were given extremely high doses over a six-month period, the animals showed excellent tolerance to the extract, with only mild kidney and liver damage, and no damage to the fetus in pregnant animals.[6]

# Observation Studies on Side Effects

Commission E states that there are no side effects known. However, they do state the following: "Extended intake can cause a temporary yellow discoloration of skin, hair, and nails. In this case, further applications of this drug must be discontinued. In rare cases, allergic skin reactions can occur. Also, accommodative disturbances, such as enlargement of the pupils and disturbances of oculomotor equilibrium, have been described." Because of the extensive clinical use of kava in Germany, researchers were able to do large-scale, multi-center surveys on the occurrence of side effects. The results of three such "observation studies" were encouraging.

In one study of 4,049 patients who took 105 mg daily of 70% kavalactones (74 mg; a relatively small daily dose) for seven weeks, the incidence of side effects—all mild and reversible—was only 1.5%.[7]

Another study of 3,029 patients taking 800 mg per day of 30% kavapyrones (240 mg; slightly above the average daily dose) over four weeks, showed a 2.3% incidence of side effects, with nine cases of allergic reaction, 31 cases of gastrointestinal discomfort, and 22 cases of headache or dizziness.[8, 9]

A study of 1,673 patients taking 800 mg, 30% kavapyrones (240 mg) for five weeks, showed an incidence of 1.7% side effects; all mild. In addition, there was significant improvement in their symptoms—anxiety, irritability, stress, sleep disorders, menopausal problems, and muscle tension.[10]

One study of 18 undergraduate volunteers at a university in New Zealand tested alertness, memory, and reaction time after consumption of a preparation of fresh kava. The results found no significant effects on these functions from the kava, even at double the doses typically consumed by South Pacific Islanders. The study concluded that kava "appears preferable to alcohol as a beverage to be consumed on social occasions, at least in terms of its effects on human performance."[11]

In the largest and longest-running study conducted to date, the six-month, 101-person study, those taking 70 mg three times daily had negligible side effects.[12] Five subjects reported a total of six unpleasant side effects, while nine of the placebo patients reported 15 total adverse effects. As we noted earlier (see Chapter 7), this is fairly remarkable—the placebo group had more side effects! Furthermore, laboratory tests showed no abnormalities in blood cells or chemistry, including kidney or liver function. Blood pressure and heart rate also remained stable or decreased slightly over the course of the study. The researcher concluded that "in contrast to both benzodiazepines and antidepressants, kava possesses an excellent side-effect profile."[13]

A number of other studies, already discussed in Chapter 7, showed similar findings in terms of side effects, and showed no adverse reactions caused by kava.[14, 15]

# Skin Rash

Known medically as "kava dermopathy," a dry, scaly, yellow skin condition was observed among some native kava drinkers as far back as the late eighteenth century. The rash occurs with long-term (months to years) high-dose kava use, estimated to be in excess of 400 mg kavalactones per day. In some Pacific Island societies, the skin condition was considered a sign of royalty because it signified that an individual had the ability to sit around all day drinking kava. Researchers initially thought that the dermopathy might be related to a kava-induced niacin deficiency or pellagra, but niacin supplements did not correct the condition. The rash clears up when kava intake is stopped.[16]

More current thinking attributes this condition to an allergic reaction or interference of kava with lipid (fat) metabolism. Whatever the cause, you needn't worry about it, since kava dermopathy has never been observed in medicinal kava users, likely due to the difference in dose. For example, the recommended dose of kava is 70 to 210 mg, while a typical half shell of coconut contains 250 mg, and several shells are consumed at a sitting. Also, the cause may be other ingredients that are found only in the fresh drink.[17] There have been no reported cases of the rash in the West, nor are any anticipated. On the other hand, my experience has taught me that biochemical individuality, allergies, and deficiencies can lead to a variety of problems.

Another side effect observed among heavy kava drinkers is an occasional state of apathy, which manifests itself as a general lethargy and loss of appetite. Again, cessation or reduction in kava consumption immediately reverses the symptoms. As Lebot, Merlin, and Lindstrom note in their book, "If kava—chewed or pounded, fresh or dried—

is drunk in moderation, it has no toxic consequences or other deleterious side effects."[18]

# Visual Effects

There are anecdotal reports that kava causes temporary changes in vision. That is, it may be possible to drink kava till you can't see straight! Researchers Garner and Klinger at the University of Auckland, New Zealand, tested a 30-year-old man who had never taken kava. They gave him 600 mg of fresh native drink (almost 10 times the normal clinical dose) on an empty stomach, with the following results:

- A reduced near point of accommodation and convergence (i.e., he had a change in the distance at which he could focus on near objects)

- Dilated pupils, similar to response to stimulants

- A disturbance of oculomotor balance; his balance, based on visual cues, was off

- No change in refractive error, visual acuity (changes in more distant viewing), or stereo acuity (3-dimensional vision that helps us locate objects spatially)

- The changes cleared up after 90 minutes

An earlier study using 800 mg of the kavalactones, dl-methysticin and dl-ethysicin, showed no change in pupillary size.[19]

This is an interesting look at seeing, or more generally, a look at kava's actions on the central nervous system. Don't worry, though. Considering the high dose (600 mg), the source (native drink), and the number of subjects (one), these findings likely have no practical bearing on the usual use of kava, which is how most individuals use it.[20]

# Tolerance, Habituation, and Withdrawal

Unlike the benzodiazepines, with kava there is no development of tolerance, habituation, or withdrawal effects. Tolerance refers to the need for increasing amounts of a substance over time to gain the same effect. This is validated by the results of various clinical studies, which varied from 4 to 25 weeks in length.[21, 22, 23]

In a 1991 Australian study, kava did not produce tolerance in mice when given at a minimally effective daily dose for seven weeks. A considerably higher dose caused partial tolerance. Learned tolerance was also not evident after three weeks of daily dosing. The implications of this for human use are that tolerance is highly unlikely.[24]

All of the research so far indicates that tolerance to kava (the requirement for ever-greater doses to achieve the same effect) does not occur, nor do any physical withdrawal symptoms. There is no impairment in mental function, including reaction time, memory, and alertness, as is associated with benzodiazepine use (see Chapter 8).

# Potential for Abuse/Addiction

As one might expect with any mind-altering substance that makes its users feel good, the question arises: Can one become a kava addict? Nineteenth and early twentieth century European explorers and missionaries thought so, but their reports of kava abuse must be taken with a rather large grain of salt. According to William Gunn in 1914, ". . . the drunkard from kava is intoxicated head to foot, body and mind. Though never hilarious or pugnacious, he is bleary-eyed, staggeringly, helplessly, disgustingly drunk. . . ."[25] Modern researchers have found little evidence to support these claims, with Lebot going so far as to say that chemical addiction to kava doesn't exist.

# The Contemporary Case
# of the Aborigines

In the early 1980s, Australian aboriginal leaders visiting Fiji and Polynesia saw how their Pacific neighbors used kava as a safe, locally grown, relaxing beverage. These leaders came back to Australia and advocated the use of kava in aboriginal communities as an alcohol substitute. Kava was enthusiastically adopted, especially in Arnhem Land in Northern Australia. It became a substance of abuse for some aboriginal users, who consumed 50 times the amount of kava habitually drunk in other regions of the South Pacific—the equivalent of several gallons of kava a day.[26]

Health problems among these kava drinkers such as malnutrition, liver damage, and shortness of breath, were widespread, leading to many sensationalistic reports in the Australian media calling for kava's abolition.[27] But other observers call the Australian reports seriously flawed, and point out that the aboriginal population in question was poverty-stricken and in poor health to begin with. If they continue to drink alcohol too, it brings up the question of whether or not kava is potentiating the toxicity in the alcohol.

"The individuals drinking the most kava were found to be in the poorest health. This is not the type of study that could be expected to accurately reflect the health effects of chronicling short-term kava use by healthy individuals," says Steven Dentali. And as Lebot, Merlin, and Lindstrom point out in their book, the Pacific Island natives where kava drinking has been common for centuries show no adverse health effects, aside from the occasional skin problems described earlier.

# Kava and Dopamine: A Note of Caution

Some kava users have found the herb's antispasmodic and muscle-relaxing actions to be useful in calming the tremors associated with Parkinson's disease and other Parkinson's-like syndromes. However, the findings of several German neurologists may give them pause.[28] In a letter to the editor, these doctors observed four patients who caused them concern:

- A 28-year-old man had sharp spasms in the muscles of his neck and eyes that began about 90 minutes after taking 100 mg of kava extract. The spasms lasted about 40 minutes.

- A 22-year-old woman experienced a similar reaction to the same product and was not taking any other medication; as did a 63-year-old woman who had taken 150 mg of kava extract three times daily for four days to treat anxiety.

- Finally, a 76-year-old woman with early signs of Parkinson's disease reported a pronounced increase in the duration and number of episodes of impaired movement after switching from pharmaceuticals to 150 mg of kava extract, which she took twice a day.

They conclude by advising caution regarding the use of kava extracts to treat patients, especially elderly ones, with Parkinson's or other conditions that result from impaired activity of dopamine, a stimulating neurotransmitter (see Chapter 3 for an explanation of neurotransmitters).

The symptoms described by the patients were those of acute dystonia, a medical term for a severe type of muscle spasm involving the neck, limbs, or tongue. It is a frequent side effect of the major tranquilizers (also called neuroleptics) such as thorazine, which are thought to work by blocking the action of dopamine. This would suggest that kava may have a similar action; blocking dopamine to cause that same dystonia.

My own hypothesis is that the occurrence of dystonia, or so-called "extrapyramidal symptoms" (EPS) may have other implications. The kava may, in fact, be unmasking or indicating a specific nutritional deficiency that shows up only when the dopamine system is stressed in this way (i.e., by the administration of a neuroleptic or kava). This suggests that kava may stress the dopamine system. If true, it might potentiate the dystonic effects of the neuroleptic, another reason to avoid such a combination. Of course, any such reactions call for immediate withdrawal of the offending substance, in this case, kava. However, as an orthomolecular psychiatrist, I am intrigued by this response, and would like to follow these findings with a look at the metabolic pathways taken by kava in the area of the brain affected in Parkinson's disease, the *basal ganglia.* This research could also potentially yield information useful in the prevention and/or treatment of such movement disorders.

Based on these cases, I cannot give a more educated opinion as to the use of kava in Parkinson's disease. I know that many physicians and herbalists have used kava successfully in these cases, and perhaps the best advice to laypeople and health practitioners alike is to be extremely cautious, with appropriately close monitoring. We still have much to learn about kava and its safe uses. The expanding use of herbal medicines in this country is new, and not covered adequately enough in our medical literature. It is up to those of us that are prescribing, teaching, and writing about them to be a clearinghouse for this information, and to disseminate information about the appropriate interventions, if known. The best advice is to err on the side of caution and do not combine kava with substances acting on the central nervous system.

In the next chapter, we'll cover combinations of other herbs and how they work with kava.

## CHAPTER 12

# Herbal
# Combinations

There are no "magic bullets," kava included. I often recommend kava in combination with other herbs and supplements. Like herbs, we are a part of nature, so these natural remedies are often best for what ails us and are most effective when used as close to their natural form as possible. This means using whole extracts rather than isolated "active ingredients." Similarly, herbs work together synergistically, enhancing each other's healing effects. Besides kava, there is a wealth of other herbs that help bring us balance in mind, body, and spirit. Kava is especially effective when used in combination with other herbs. At the end of the chapter, we summarize a new study showing the positive effects of one such combination.

In cases of mixed anxiety and depression, for example, I often use St. John's wort. For insomnia, I often add valerian, hops, and passion flower, among others. Ginkgo is particularly helpful in older patients who are having problems with memory and concentration. There are also the adapto-gens for overall regulation and balance—ginseng, ashwa-ganda, suma, and reishi mushroom.

These herbal mixtures are usually given along with a va-riety of vitamins, minerals, and other supplements specifically tailored to the individual to support his or her body chem-istry. Other nutrients that support the adrenal glands—which are often depleted by stress, anxiety, and depression—are vit-amin C, magnesium, zinc, and the B vitamins. I give all my patients a high potency vitamin-mineral formula supplying the basic nutrients that are often inadequate in our diets. Ex-cept when I want to test for specific effects or sensitivities, I seldom prescribe single herbs or supplements. There are ex-cellent resources for learning more about herbs, some of which are listed in Appendix B.

## St. John's Wort (*Hypericum perforatum*)

Stress and anxiety are closely related to depression, and in fact, many people who suffer from depression also must cope with anxiety. About half the patients with anxiety or panic disorders develop a major depression within five years. It has been esti-mated that 18 million Americans suffer from depression. This is not the brief fluctuation in mood that comes from a bad day at the office, but an ongoing, debilitating medical illness. De-pressed people often feel fatigued, empty, and hopeless. They may lose interest in the things that normally provide pleasure, including social and sexual activity. With the use of appropri-ate nutritional supplements, depression can often be treated without medication. In the absence of treatment, on the other hand, clinically depressed individuals can become immersed in a self-perpetuating negative spiral.

Research has shown that the centuries-old herb St. John's wort is as effective for mild to moderate depression as pre-scription antidepressants such as Prozac, but without the

side effects. In addition, no one has ever died from an overdose of St. John's wort, while for every 1 million prescriptions of antidepressants, 30 people die each year of over-
doses. For the past five years, St. John's wort has been the
treatment of choice in much of Europe, Germany in particular, outnumbering all antidepressant drug prescriptions at
least 10 to 1, likely more. It is used successfully to treat sea-
sonal affective disorder (SAD), anxiety, premenstrual syndrome (PMS), and insomnia. In the words of one happy
user, ". . . I feel like a veil has been lifted. I am sleeping better, dreaming more, and remembering my dreams!" And according to another, "It was never like this on Prozac. I'm
more energetic and focused, and there's more laughter."

## Actions

Many sources have warned about a "tyramine" or "cheese effect" with St. John's wort, necessitating certain food restric-
tions. Based on further evidence, these warnings have proven
unnecessary. St. John's wort likely acts as a serotonin re-uptake
inhibitor, similar to Prozac, and may also have an enhancing
action on the stimulant neurotransmitters, dopamine and
norepinephrine. In vitro (test tube) studies also indicate an
affinity for the GABA neural receptors. These are the ones affected by the benzodiazepines, which would explain St. John's
wort antianxiety effects.

## Advantages Compared to Antidepressant Drugs

As we have already said, a great advantage of herbs over the
targeted "magic bullet" effects of synthetic drugs is that herbs
are complex combinations of many ingredients with multiple
actions. This often increases the beneficial effects while reducing possible side effects (but, with anything else, with
some exceptions). Antidepressants, on the other hand, have
a variety of side effects, including headaches, nausea, sexual
dysfunction, insomnia, sedation, agitation, heart arrhythmias,
weight changes, rashes, and short-term memory loss.

St. John's wort is nonaddictive, nonhabituating, and has no withdrawal symptoms. It does not interfere with REM sleep, enhances sleep and dreaming, has no adverse effects when mixed with alcohol or drugs (with some exceptions), and does not cause drowsiness or agitation. It also has pronounced antianxiety and anti-insomnia effects. It may actually be a natural releaser of the sleep-regulating hormone melatonin.

## Dosage

The average recommended dose is 300 mg of standardized extract (0.3% hypericin) two to three times daily, in tablets, capsules, or tincture, depending on individual preference. It can take from one to several weeks for the full effect to occur, though I have seen it work almost immediately. These guidelines are general, and results vary depending on the patient and particular combination.

## Research

The *British Medical Journal* published a review of 23 controlled studies involving 1,757 depressed patients. The results showed that St. John's wort is three times more effective than a placebo and as effective as prescription antidepressants, but without their side effects. In a landmark occurrence, the National Institute of Mental Health is launching a $4.3 million study based at Duke University Medical Center to test the herb's effectiveness in treating depression. The medical establishment is clearly taking notice of herbal medicine—the start of an exciting and much-needed trend.[1]

## St. John's Wort with Kava

I will often give St. John's wort in combination with kava, due to the complementary effects they have on depression, anxiety, and insomnia. Unlike St. John's wort, which may not begin taking effect for a week or two, or even longer, kava works immediately. There are a number of excellent products on the market that combine the two.

Herbalist Ed Smith had the following story to tell about the use of his St. John's wort/kava tincture (35% St. John's wort, 30% kava, 25% skullcap, 10% prickly ash): "An engineer I know came to see me. He had a serious history of depression, and had even attempted suicide twice over the years. None of the conventional therapies were helping. Then he started taking this combination. Three months later he called me with an enthusiasm I'd never heard before, saying, 'My life has changed completely. I look at the guy smiling back at me in the mirror, and I don't recognize him. It's given me a new lease on life!' A year later, by the way, the man was still taking these herbs and doing well."

Given the uncertainty regarding the exact actions of kava and St. John's wort, some experts, such as Dr. Don Brown, director of Natural Products Research Consultants in Seattle, remain wary about using the two together. However, there have been no reported problems in the United States or in Germany, where these are taken under medical supervision. There may be those who are allergic or hypersensitive to one of the herbs or the combination. If the reaction hasn't been serious, I suggest that the person take each product separately and observe the response before combining them again.

## Herbs for Insomnia

### *Valerian* (Valeriana officinalis)

Insomnia is another serious problem, affecting 43% of the population (see Chapter 9). Valerian extract, a folk remedy derived from the dried rhizomes and roots of the plant, has been used for centuries as a natural tranquilizer for disorders such as anxiety, insomnia, menstrual problems, exhaustion, headaches, and "nervous" stomach. Health conscious consumers in Europe and the United States are discovering that valerian root has a calming effect and helps them fall asleep more easily.

### Valerian and Kava for Insomnia

Ben was a 35-year-old automobile salesman, who asked if I could help him find a more natural approach to his long-standing insomnia. He had just completed a withdrawal program from what he called his "bedside candy store" of various sleeping medications. He had disliked his dependence on them. Besides, he found that unless he switched them around regularly, they would cease to work. He'd been off the medications for about a month, and had been taking valerian as a bedtime substitute. He fell asleep easily, but found that he would wake up after several hours, unable to fall back to sleep.

I suggested that he add kava, both during the day and at bedtime. The result? He experienced an extended, deep, satisfying night's sleep, with none of the "hangover" that he experienced on the drugs. Besides being less irritable and more relaxed during the day, he noticed that he was able to think more clearly than ever. He described the kava as "turning off the tape in his head"—that constant inner chatter that had interfered with both his sleep and clear thinking.

---

Valerian is often included in sleeping preparations along with a number of other herbs, including kava. I added the kava, because while valerian helps induce sleep, kava helps improve the duration and quality. A Swiss study found it better than placebo.[2] A German study comparing the benzodiazepine Halcion to valerian plus lemonbalm yielded the same sleep results, but without the drug's hangover, loss of concentration, and addictiveness.[3, 4] Also, like St John's wort, it poses no danger when combined with alcohol. The recommended dose is 50 to 100 mg taken two to three times daily, and 150 to 300 mg taken 45 minutes before bedtime, using a standardized dose of 0.8% valeric acid.

Valerian is useful in withdrawal from benzodiazepines, since both may act on the GABA receptors in the brain (see Chapter 3). With prolonged use at higher doses, it can cause morning hangovers and headaches. I prefer using it in smaller doses, in combination with kava and other herbs. As mentioned earlier, I have used this combination while helping patients withdraw from benzodiazepines, but cannot recommend it to others until further research is conducted (see Chapter 5). In any case, it is certainly useful as a replacement once the withdrawal is complete.

## *Hops* (Humulus lupulus)

Hops have been used for centuries as a mild sedative and sleeping aid. Hops' primary use is to calm nerves and induce sleep, usually in combination with other herbal sedatives such as passion flower, valerian root, and skullcap. Its sedative action works directly on the central nervous system. The dose is around 200 mg per day, but varies with the combination.

## *Passion Flower* (Passiflora incarnata)

Passion flower's mild sedative effect has been well-substantiated in numerous animal and human studies. The herb encourages deep, restful, uninterrupted sleep, with no side effects. Passion flower has been commonly used in the treatment of concentration problems in school children and as a sedative for the elderly. Dosage varies with the combination, but is generally 100 to 200 mg per day of standardized product.

## Herb Combinations for Insomnia

Yolanda was a 20-year-old college junior, who was enrolled in a pre-med program with a demanding course load. As if that weren't enough, she balanced her academic career with a job at a restaurant, and an intense relationship. The result: Yolanda was stressed, nervous, and had trouble sleeping. She described being constantly tired, irritable, having trouble concentrating in class, and suffering from aching legs and back pain.

My herbal remedy for Yolanda consisted of kava during the day, once or twice as needed, and in a combination formula with valerian and passion flower at night. They worked together harmoniously for the desired effects—tension relief, sound restful sleep, enhanced concentration, and a positive mood. Inspired by her own experience, she hopes to go on to become a practitioner of complementary medicine.

---

### *Other Sleep Remedies*

There are also many other helpful herbal sleep remedies. Here are some combinations from master Herbalist Christopher Hobbs:

- Basic formula: passion flower, valerian, and California poppy
- Insomnia plus anxiety: California poppy, hawthorne (a heart tonic), and hops
- Anti-stress mixture: two parts each of chamomile, lavender, lemon balm, and linden, with one part orange peel[5]

# Adaptogens to the Rescue

---

It is clear that herbs do not distinguish between physical and mental symptoms and that most herbs affect the mind and body in a great variety of ways. Our allopathic, linear way of looking at symptoms and treatments can never be as sophisticated, or as successful, as these healers from nature.

## Ginseng: A Family of Adaptogens

The major forms of the well-known family of herbs called ginseng—Korean, American, and Siberian—are all regarded as adaptogens. Adaptogens work by achieving a balancing effect in the human body to restore or counter the effects of stress. I will focus on only one of them, Siberian ginseng, which is not actually a ginseng at all. Nonetheless, it is an excellent adaptogen and works well with other herbs.

Siberian ginseng, or eleuthero, is a tall shrub that grows in the wild in the Far East. It is used as a remedy for stress, fatigue, anxiety, and depression, with no harmful long-term effects. It has also proved effective in improving intellectual performance and enhancing mental stamina. The Russians have been far ahead of us in their recognition of this valuable herb, with their athletes taking it for months before the Olympics. Cosmonauts likewise remain alert and energetic, despite the physical and mental stress of life in space. Research has shown specific effects that support the central nervous system, liver, circulatory system, immune, and hormonal systems. In particular, ginseng supports and replenishes the adrenal glands, an essential part of our stress-fighting system that often becomes depleted in those suffering from anxiety and depression.

### Effective Results from Ginseng

Melissa was a 40-year-old actress with a 10-month history of chronic fatigue syndrome. She complained that she would collapse in a heap after only 15 minutes of light exercise and would have to rest for an hour or so to recover. Her nighttime sleep was not restorative, and her body ached with fibromyalgia. I prescribed Siberian ginseng (200 mg, two to three times daily), licorice root, reishi mushroom, and kava. Within four weeks, she was sleeping well, her fibromyalgia was much improved, and she was able to exercise moderately for 30 minutes, with no fatigue.

---

## *Ashwaganda* (Withania somnifera)

An Ayurvedic herb increasingly integrated into Western herbal practice, Ashwaganda is an excellent adaptogen. It is an immune enhancer, and is both energizing and calming, handling the various aspects of stress. Similar to St. John's wort, it reduces levels of the stress hormone cortisol. The dose is 300 mg, standardized extract, two to three times daily.

## *Licorice* (Glycyrrhiza glabra)

Among other uses, licorice root provides support for the adrenal glands, helping with mild adrenal insufficiency and hypoglycemia, as in Melissa's case. It is also used in women for its estrogen-balancing properties. In the words of natural hormone pioneer Dr. Jonathan Wright, "Licorice is like hamburger helper for estrogen." It stimulates the adrenal cortex directly to produce mineral corticoids, glucocorticoids, and adrenal sex hormones, then prevents breakdown of these hormones by the liver and kidneys. It helps to raise low blood pressure, which often accompanies chronic fatigue, but it can also lead to hypertension (high blood pressure) in susceptible individuals. To avoid this side effect, the deglycyrrhinized form is used in many instances, such as in treating ulcers, but then the hormonal effect is lost.

## *Reishi Mushroom* (Ganodermum lucidum)

A host of other natural substances possess stress fighting properties as well and are often used to modify or enhance the effects of other herbs. Among them is the Chinese reishi mushroom, which has multiple benefits and no significant side effects. Similar to kava, reishi also helps to calm anxiety. I have also had great success using kava with reishi for treatment of chronic fatigue syndrome and fibromyalgia, as with Melissa. The average dose is 250 mg, two to three times daily. St. John's wort has also been effective in alleviating symptoms of fibromyalgia.

## *Ginkgo Biloba* (Ginkgo biloba)

Of the many debilitating side effects of chronic stress, decreased brain function is one of the most serious. Fortunately, the popular extract of the ginkgo biloba tree provides an excellent antidote. One of the oldest living species of tree, it is often called a "living fossil." The Chinese have long used ginkgo fruit for lung ailments and cardiovascular diseases, and recently Western researchers have been studying the ginkgo biloba leaf as a treatment for senility and circulation problems. Ginkgo is especially effective for improving mental acuity in the elderly, while its circulation- and neurological-enhancing properties have benefits for adults of all ages. The usual dose is 120 to 160 mg daily in two or three divided doses.

### Ginkgo Biloba Aids the Elderly

One beneficiary of ginkgo was George, a 63-year-old recently retired engineer. Feeling old, replaced in his high-power position by the next generation, and finding his memory and mental acuity beginning to fail, George was depressed, tense, and irritable. He insisted he needed alcohol to help him with his insomnia. His concerned wife reported that he was drinking more and making love less and insisted he come to see me.

I prescribed an herbal regimen that combined kava for sleep and anxiety, along with ginkgo for mental functioning. I added ginseng and reishi for balance and wild oats (*Aveena sativa*) for calming and sexual enhancement. I also added milk thistle (silymarin) to support his liver, which was taxed by the alcohol.

The results over the next month were impressive. The kava helped George to lower his inner stress levels and relax, while the ginkgo helped sharpen his acuity and give him the focus he needed. Even his libido took an upswing, likely due to the stress relief, wild oats, and ginkgo. Together with their adaptogenic functions, the other herbs supported his long overstressed adrenals. His wife was pleased, to say the least.

---

## Other Combinations

Terry Willard has been combining kava with ginger and cayenne in the form of Flex-Herb, which he calls "massage in a bottle." This creates an excellent muscle relaxant, especially in conjunction with chiropractic adjustment.

Skullcap (*Scutellaria lateriflora*) is highly regarded by Ed Smith of HerbPharm. "Skullcap is one of my favorites," Smith says. "It's not well-known, but I've used it for years. It acts as what I call a neurological adaptogen, in the way it boosts the proper working of the nervous system.

"Another good one is oat seed extract, which has been used in India for centuries as a treatment for opium addiction, and also acts to bolster the nervous system."

As you can see, different healers have their own favorite herbs and often create mixtures of two or more; the proportions calibrated for the individual being treated. More exciting still is the fact that these herbs, along with other natural stress treatments, can be used as a complement to kava. Indeed, when used with kava in an integrated program to treat stress, anxiety, and insomnia, these therapies can prove far more effective together than if used separately.

# A Promising New Study
# on a Kava Combination

Nirbhay Singh and Cynthia Ellis have completed an as-yet un-published study on the use of a kava combination for stress and anxiety.[6, 7] Singh's brother, researcher Yadhu Singh, is mentioned several times in this book for his excellent work in this field.[8, 9] Raised in Fiji, both have had personal as well as professional experience with the herb.

There are at least three significant things to point out about this study, which make it particularly relevant to the stressful lifestyles we are all living:

- It was measuring the effect of these herbs on stress as well as anxiety

- It involved a "normal," non-patient population

- It was done in the United States

The study examined a combination product: 60 mg of kava, plus a synergistic group of herbs also known to promote relax-ation—passion flower, chamomile, hops, and schizandra.

Sixty self-selected volunteers with elevated stress and anxiety levels took part in the study. They had been re-cruited through ads in health food stores, pharmacies, and supermarkets and were not a "patient" population. Half of the group took a twice-daily dose of the kava combination product (60 mg × 2 = 120 mg of kava) and half took the placebo. This was a "double-blind" study; that is, neither the researchers nor the subjects knew which kind the partici-pants were given.

Their anxiety (State-Trait Anxiety Inventory) and stress levels (Daily Stress Inventories) were measured, before, during (three times), and at the end of the study, for a total of five measurements. Those taking the kava product experienced a significant decrease in both their stress and anxiety scores, with greater improvement over time, while the placebo group did not experience such a decrease.

According to the authors, this is the first study to show that kava reduces stress associated with the daily hassles of life. Moreover, this reduction in stress and anxiety increased with time; the longer they were on the product, the better they felt. And there were no side effects. The findings are consistent with other research and anecdotal data, as well as my own clinical experience with kava and its combinations.

Research considerations:

- Since this study has not been published, it has yet to undergo "peer-review," the critical professional appraisal and analysis of its method and results.

- The study reports almost no change in the placebo group, an unusual occurrence in anxiety studies. On the other hand, at least one German kava study had a similar finding (see Chapter 8).

- Nowhere in the article is it mentioned that the product tested contains active herbal ingredients—other than kava—that are known by themselves to produce relaxation. In fact, the study's positive findings more correctly apply to this specific combination, rather than to kava itself. But, why stress about it?

The results of this preliminary study are promising, and we look forward to much more American research of this kind.

# Conclusion

As you can see, kava is often used along with other herbs and supplements. Despite its use in combinations in the traditional medicine of the islands, it is a relative newcomer to the West. We are just discovering its alchemy with other, more familiar herbs. The proof of an herb's efficacy is in how it does clinically, no matter how good it looks in theory. We've touched on some of the kava combinations that I have found most effective. Next we will look at how to create a healthy lifestyle program that supports mind, body, and spirit.

## CHAPTER 13

# Diet and Supplements

You are what you eat.

—*Robert Crumb,* Mr. Natural

I n an ideal world, our food would supply us with the nutrients we require. However, the average American diet is already deficient in many of our essential nutrients. We
need only consider the common diet of high-sugar, low-fiber,
chemically preserved foods that many people consume on a
regular basis. In addition, such poor nutrition often leads
to impaired absorption of nutrients, since the very ones
needed to promote a healthy digestive system are often lack-
ing. This can create a vicious cycle of ever-increasing deficiency, and yet further breakdown of digestive function.

Even if we improve our eating habits, though, food
alone will not be sufficient for a majority of us. Our food supply may be significantly low in micronutrients compared to

the same foods a generation ago. This is due to many foods being grown in depleted soils, and the use of chemical fertilizers. Then, no matter how nutrient-rich the original product was, refining, processing, freezing, and even exposure to air all take their toll in the depletion of essential nutrients. Furthermore, each individual has his or her own nutritional requirements, some of which may exceed the amount that could possibly be ingested from even the healthiest of diets.

As a nation, we are at once overfed and undernourished, and a poorly nourished body contains a malnourished brain. Like many other ailments of the mind and body, stress and anxiety can be exacerbated, or even caused by, nutritional imbalance. Stress, too, draws on our nutrient storehouse. For example:

- The kidneys tend to retain sodium at the expense of potassium, thereby producing a potassium deficiency

- Calcium and magnesium are withdrawn from the bone matrix, encouraging the development of osteoporosis or bone thinning

- B vitamins and magnesium are depleted during the body's biochemical response to stress. This alone can contribute to many of the disorders associated with stress, including anxiety and depression

Balance can often be restored through the appropriate use of vitamins, minerals, and amino acids. As a result, I recommend a high potency vitamin-mineral supplement for my patients, as well as extra amounts of certain nutrients based on symptoms.

# Vitamins: Vital Nutrients for Combating Stress and Supporting Mental Health

Vitamins and minerals are cofactors and catalysts in our metabolic functions and have far-reaching effects on our health.

The B vitamins, for example, play a vital role in cellular energy. Our bodies cannot create vitamins, so a well-balanced, supplemented diet is necessary to obtain adequate amounts of these essential nutrients. There is growing evidence that some of these micronutrients help prevent illnesses, including cancer. The antioxidants such as vitamins C, E, and beta-carotene are considered major players in this regard. Vitamins act as catalytic agents in the body, helping to speed up the chemical processes that are vital for both survival and brain function. As mentioned, they are depleted by stress, which can result in anxiety, irritability, and depression. Fortunately, these can be corrected with supplementation.

The Recommended Daily Allowance (RDA) is widely believed to be inadequate. These figures are based on the minimal requirements for prevention of severe deficiency disease, rather than on the requirements for optimum health or deficiency correction. My recommendations, which exceed the RDA, are for formulas containing vitamins B1, B3, and B6; 50 mg daily, with higher doses for people with specific disorders.

## Vitamin B Complex

This is a group of water-soluble vitamins that work together to support many metabolic processes, and consists of thiamin, riboflavin, niacin, pantothenic acid, pyridoxine, cobalamin, pangamic acid, biotin, choline, folic acid, inositol, and PABA (para-aminobenzoic acid).

The B vitamins perform the following key functions in the body:

- Thiamin ($B_1$): Converts glucose (blood sugar) into fuel. Without it the brain runs out of energy, causing fatigue, depression, irritability, and anxiety. Deficiencies can also cause problems with memory, sleep, and digestion. Refined carbohydrates—devoid of their natural B vitamin content—deplete the body's $B_1$ supply.

- Riboflavin ($B_2$): Helps in conversion of amino acids into neurotransmitters. Deficiency may occur in dairy-free diets.

- Vitamin $B_3$ (niacin): Pellagra, which produces diarrhea, dermatitis, and dementia, is caused by niacin deficiency. Deficiencies of vitamin $B_3$ can also produce agitation and anxiety, as well as mental and physical slowness, all reversible with megadose supplementation.

- Pantothenic acid ($B_5$): Supports adrenal function and is essential in times of stress.

- Vitamin $B_6$ (pyridoxine): An essential cofactor in making neurotransmitters, it is useful for treating premenstrual syndrome (PMS) and carpal tunnel syndrome. There is a strong correlation between vitamin $B_6$ deficiency and depression. Deficiencies can be caused by malabsorption diseases and certain drugs, including MAOI antidepressants (see Chapter 5) and birth control pills. I recommend that all women on birth control pills take 50 mg of vitamin $B_6$ daily.

- Cobalamin ($B_{12}$): $B_{12}$ is important for the nervous system and the metabolism of protein, fats, and carbohydrates. It may be poorly absorbed by the elderly, causing symptoms of depression, fatigue, and even dementia. I have found $B_{12}$ injections or tablets that dissolve under the tongue, together with folic acid, to be extremely helpful in these cases. It can also boost mood and energy in chronic fatigue syndrome patients.

- Inositol: Found in lecithin, along with choline, is essential for the functioning of the central nervous system.

- Folic acid (folate): Folic acid assists in the creation of many neurotransmitters. It is also essential to the production of hemoglobin, the oxygen-bearing substance in red blood cells. Pregnant women are routinely prescribed a folic acid supplement to prevent spinal cord defects. Alcoholism, and various drugs, including aspirin, birth control pills, barbiturates, and anticonvulsants deplete folic acid. It is usually administered along with vitamin $B_{12}$ since a folic acid deficiency can mask a $B_{12}$ deficiency.

### *Vitamin C* (Ascorbic Acid)

These are the significant properties of vitamin C:

- Antioxidant: Works together with vitamins A, E, and others to counteract the effects of *free radicals,* the supercharged molecular fragments that destroy tissue

- Antidepressant: Deficiencies can produce depression, which is often one of the first signs of vitamin C deficiency.[1] One preliminary study showed that a single three-gram dose of vitamin C reduced symptoms by 40% in 11 manic and 12 depressed patients after only four hours

- Antistress nutrient: During times of stress, urinary excretion of vitamin C is increased[2]

Other important factors about vitamin C are:

- Stress, pregnancy, and lactation increase the body's need for vitamin C

- Aspirin, tetracycline, and birth control pills can deplete the body's supply

- A good maintenance dose is one to three grams daily; with more for people with stress and anxiety, smokers, and those exposed to toxins

# Minerals

There are at least 15 minerals that are essential to health. Inadequate intake can lead to mental and behavioral problems,

including stress and anxiety, often before any physical symptoms appear. The most important minerals are calcium, magnesium, phosphorus, iron, iodine, zinc, chromium, potassium,
manganese, selenium, copper, vanadium, and boron.

We will discuss the key minerals here, but be aware that
research clearly indicates the importance of the other minerals or "trace elements." For example, research has shown
that selenium is an excellent protection against cancer.[3]

### Sodium and Potassium

These minerals are considered together because they regulate cellular fluid levels by reciprocal balance. With the excessive salt (sodium) intake in the American diet, the typical
American has an unhealthy ratio of sodium to potassium of
2:1. This can lead to water retention, with such symptoms as
high blood pressure, PMS, and anxiety and depression. The
recommended ratio is reversed at least a 5:1 ratio of potassium to sodium. Most fruits and vegetables have a ratio of
100:1, so you can see how far off we are and how important
these minerals are to our diets, especially under times of
stress. Potassium need is increased by alcohol, sugar, tea,
coffee, most common diuretic drugs, and stress. The adrenals require adequate potassium to do their jobs; at least
three to five grams daily. Potassium-rich foods include ba-
nanas, oranges, potatoes, and carrots.

### Iron

Iron deficiency can result in anemia—remember the old
Geritol commercial "some call it tired blood"? This can show
up as anxiety or depression, irritability, fatigue, loss of attention span, and insomnia. Iron deficiency is easily diagnosed
by a blood test. One study found that nearly half of all pre-
menopausal women and one-third of all children do not get
enough iron, so supplementation in these groups could have
a significant impact on the frequency of depression and

other disorders. On the other hand, excessive iron can lead to toxicity, especially in men, who are not losing the mineral regularly through menstruation. Thus, men shouldn't supplement with iron without medical supervision.

## Calcium, Magnesium, and Boron

These minerals offer protection against osteoporosis. Taken at bedtime, the combination of calcium and magnesium promotes natural, healthy sleep. Taking large doses of calcium without magnesium can deplete magnesium and actually promote osteoporosis and other problems associated with magnesium deficiency. Magnesium is deficient in most diets and is depleted by stress. An anti-stress mineral, it guards against depression, is necessary for calcium and vitamin C metabolism, and helps convert glucose into energy. Alcohol increases the body's requirement for this mineral. Several studies, and my own experience, have shown that magnesium injections can bring relief from symptoms such as fatigue, aches and pains, weakness, lethargy, migraine headaches, PMS, panic disorder, and allergies. The usual 2:1 ratio of calcium to magnesium in supplements may be incorrect for many, since there are more sources of calcium than magnesium in most diets. My recommendation is generally a 1:1 supplementation.

## Zinc

Zinc serves many important functions. First, it is essential to brain function. In addition to irritability, mental slowness, and emotional disorders, zinc deficiency can produce changes in taste, smell, and appetite, reduced immune function, and rough skin. Zinc is an immune stimulant and promotes healing. It is an excellent treatment for anorexia and bulimia in high doses. Zinc is essential in hormone formation, and adolescents who are deficient can develop acne. Older men should take it to prevent prostate enlargement.

## Essential Fatty Acids

---

These are necessary for many chemical processes within the body. Omega-6 fatty acids are found in vegetable oils such as grape seed, borage, and evening primrose. Flax and fish oils, found in fatty coldwater fish such as mackerel and salmon, provide the omega-3 fatty acids, especially DHA, which is essential for brain function. Fish really is brain food! The essential fatty acids are the building blocks for the nervous system. They support the immune system, fight inflammation, and support the activity of neurotransmitters (including serotonin) and steroid hormones (including the sex hormones).

# Amino Acids

---

Anxiety and depression can result from a deficiency of brain messengers called neurotransmitters. Amino acids, the building blocks of protein, are the precursors, or raw materials, for neurotransmitters and other mood-regulating compounds, and can be given as supplements. Since amino acids are found in such high-protein foods as meat, fish, and eggs, you might think that the way to increase your amino-acid levels would be to eat more of these foods.

However, disorders such as stress and anxiety are caused by specific amino acid imbalances, often glutamine, glycine, GABA, and taurine. Amino acids are also often used in the treatment of seizure disorders, drug and alcohol withdrawal symptoms, Attention Deficit Disorder (ADD), and bipolar disorder.

Deficiencies in the amino acids phenylalanine, tyrosine, and tryptophan are most directly related to depression. Phenylalanine and tyrosine produce the neurotransmitter norepinephrine, and tryptophan is converted to serotonin.

Tryptophan is available only by prescription at compounding pharmacies, i.e., pharmacies that carry natural medicines (see Appendix B). However, 5-hydroxytryptophan (5-HTP), a downstream substance in the metabolic production of trypto-phan, is now available commercially.

It is important to take sufficient amounts of the "co-factors," such as vitamin $B_6$, which your body needs to prop-erly process these amino acids. Amino acids can also be combined with herbs such as kava and St. John's wort. I rec-ommend that amino acid therapy be carried out under pro-fessional supervision, to ensure correct dosage.

### Phosphatidylserine

This is a major phospholipid in the brain that helps to en-sure proper nerve function. It enhances mood, behavior, and mental function by increasing the accumulation, stor-age, and release of several neurotransmitters.

# Macronutrients:
# A Healthy Diet for a Healthy Mind

The micronutrients—amino acids, vitamins, and minerals—are the fine-tuning elements or cofactors that help convert our food into tissue and energy. The bulk of our diet con-sists of the macronutrients—carbohydrates, proteins, and fats. Supplements, while necessary, do not take the place of an adequate diet. Following are some overall guidelines for healthy eating.

### Carbohydrates

These include cereals, grains, breads, and vegetables and are rated by their glycemic index. This index measures how quickly a specific food is turned into glucose, or blood sugar, which in turn stimulates the pancreas to release insulin. High glycemic foods, such as doughnuts and white bread, raise blood-glucose levels rapidly, resulting in a large, fast release of insulin. Insulin removes sugar from the system and stores it as fat and glycogen. This causes blood-glucose levels to drop, making us feel weak, lightheaded, and even cranky, as we see next.

# Stress and Hypoglycemia

Each individual reacts to stressors in his or her own unique way. In some people, chronic stress leads to a perpetual hyper-alertness and sensitivity, while others may go psychologically numb or sink into depression. Often, symptoms are mixed into such a complex bundle that it's nearly impossible to see that stress is actually at the root of these other problems. Many medical conditions may first appear in this way. The following case illustrates the complex interactions of mind, mood, and hormones; how these are affected by stress; and how a holistic approach can be used to diagnose and treat stress.

### An Example of Stress and the Body:
### Hypoglycemia and Adrenal Dysfunction

#### *Background*

On the surface, Kim's situation was not unlike that of many Americans today. A successful 38-year-old professional, she was a single working mother of two energetic teenagers. She had recently been promoted into a mid-level management position in a growing computer software firm and described herself as ambitious and an achiever prone to workaholic habits. Her day began with a 45-minute freeway commute, a prelude to a very stressful work day. Outside of work, she was involved in school, church, and community activities and found herself frazzled by a lack of time and confronted with a growing list of never finished tasks. She complained of extreme fatigue, lack of time for herself, and feeling guilty about not spending more time with her kids. Exhausted and near burnout, she felt stretched emotionally, financially, and professionally.

To make matters worse, Kim would awaken at 3:00 or 4:00 A.M. most mornings, her heart pounding, her mind racing, and be unable to fall back to sleep until just before the alarm rang at 6:30. It didn't matter what time she went to bed. She would fall asleep easily—or as she put it—"collapse into bed in a heap," but nothing helped the early morning awakening, including the sleeping pill temazepam (Restoril).

### Diagnosis

It would appear that Kim was suffering from a straightforward case of stress-induced fatigue, compounded by sleep deprivation. If that were so, she would not be alone. The *Annals of Internal Medicine* recently reported that one out of four people surveyed complained of fatigue lasting longer than two weeks. In fact, fatigue is now one of the most frequent reasons people call their doctors. And the incidence of insomnia among Americans is now 43%.[4] However, there were emotional components to Kim's condition: anxiety, and depression. This is not unusual, as fatigue, anxiety, and depression often coexist. Fatigue may lead to anxiety and/or depression, and vice versa. But what did these symptoms mean? Are they disease states in and of themselves or are they indicators of a deeper, underlying process?

Kim's other symptoms gave me a clue. She craved sweets, had frequent headaches and heart palpitations, and felt shaky at times. These were worse when she missed a meal, and were relieved by eating. Her symptoms pointed to hypoglycemia, which can appear in many forms: as depression, irritability, anxiety, panic attacks, fatigue, "brain fog," headaches (including migraines), insomnia, muscular weakness, and tremors. All of these symptoms may be relieved by food. A person may crave sweets, coffee, alcohol, or drugs; in fact, many addictions are related to hypoglycemia.

## Diet

Kim's hypoglycemia related to a combination of overstressed adrenal glands and poor diet. To support her adrenals and balance her blood sugar, I made the following recommendations:

First, I prescribed dietary changes, including the elimination of refined carbohydrates, such as sugar and white flour, as well as cutting out coffee and alcohol. I also recommended small, frequent meals containing protein and complex carbohydrates, which have a high glycemic index. This index measures how quickly a specific food is turned into glucose, or blood sugar, which in turn stimulates the pancreas to release insulin. When Kim ate high glycemic foods, such as doughnuts and candy, or drank coffee, her blood sugar levels rose rapidly. This led to a large, fast release of insulin which then removed the sugar from circulation, storing it as fat and glycogen. This caused her blood sugar level to drop over the next one to two hours, making Kim feel weak, lightheaded, and even cranky. When this cycle repeated itself enough, the overtaxed adrenal glands became exhausted—and so did she.

The solution for Kim was to eat foods with a low glycemic index, such as vegetables and whole grains. These are turned into glucose more slowly, allowing for more stable blood-glucose levels and greater energy levels. This helps normalize blood sugar levels, increase stamina and stress-bearing ability, and stabilize moods. Complex carbohydrates also raise serotonin levels, creating a calming, antidepressant, and antianxiety effect. Like Kim, our fast food, coffee-and-doughnuts diets create more stress in that they contribute to hypoglycemia, which impairs our ability to cope.

## Supplements

I prescribed a daily nutritional supplement regimen for Kim. This included a high potency multi-vitamin-mineral for basic support, containing at least 75 mg of each of the B vitamins and 200 mg chromium to help balance blood sugar; magnesium, 400 mg; manganese, 10 mg; potassium, 500 to 1,000 mg; zinc, 15 to 30 mg. In addition, I prescribed pantothenic acid (Vitamin $B_5$), 2 g and vitamin C, 3,000 mg. For cravings, I prescribed glutamine 500 to 1,000 mg, as needed. This is also useful for alcohol cravings, not surprising in view of the close relationship between the two conditions.

## Exercise

Kim began to exercise regularly, which allowed her to burn fats, maintain blood glucose levels, relieve anxiety, and elevate her mood. Regular exercise can actually reduce the amount of adrenal hormones the body releases in response to stress. In addition, it raises the level of the mood-elevating hormones, or endorphins, in the brain.

## Results

Kim's new habits had a marked effect on her moods, which became more stable, without the anxiety and depression. Her physical symptoms cleared. There were no more early morning awakenings, no more headaches, and no fatigue. The stresses of life as a busy mother and office worker continued, but she no longer fell victim to her internal physiology. She was better able to control her reactions from a place of inner calm, rather than as a forced behavioral change. She now had an internal buffer against stress—functioning adrenal glands and a smoother supply of blood sugar to her body—particularly to her brain.

---

Kim is not alone in her stress and hypoglycemia. The predisposition to hypoglycemia runs in families, so if you are

---

**Hypoglycemia Questionnaire**
Scoring: 0 = Never; 1 = Occasionally;
2 = Often; 3 = Most of the time

1. Experience dizziness when standing quickly      \_\_\_\_\_

2. Get irritable, weak, or shaky if meal missed      \_\_\_\_\_

3. Crave sweets      \_\_\_\_\_

4. Experience heart racing after eating sugar      \_\_\_\_\_

5. Feel tired one to three hours after a meal      \_\_\_\_\_

6. Feel faint easily      \_\_\_\_\_

7. Need coffee for energy      \_\_\_\_\_

8. Feel tired or fatigued      \_\_\_\_\_

9. Experience periods of emotional instability      \_\_\_\_\_

10. Experience headaches, relieved by eating      \_\_\_\_\_

Less than 3: Hypoglycemia is not a problem
4–9:  Hypoglycemia is likely a problem
10 and over: Hypoglycemia is definitely a problem

---

prone, you must be more conscientious in your attention to stress, diet, and nutritional supplements. The most common causes of hypoglycemia are poor eating habits and excessive stress. Notice how these factors affect you, and get with the program. Since hypoglycemia symptoms are a warning signal that an imbalance is present, it should not simply be treated with psychotherapy or antianxiety and antidepressant drugs. The immediate problem is best treated with dietary changes, supplements, and relaxation techniques. Later therapy can be helpful in revealing and dealing with the underlying dynamics.

Conventional medicine has tended not to focus on hypoglycemia, due to the difficulty of obtaining clear, objective proof of its existence. Although a three-hour "glucose tolerance test" is available for confirmation, it does not always show abnormalities with people who obviously seem to have hypoglycemia, while with other people there are no symptoms even though the test seems to be abnormal. Nonetheless, hypoglycemia definitely seems to be a problem for many people. It is best diagnosed by taking a good medical and psychological history.

Perhaps you recognize some of Kim's symptoms as your own. You can take the "Hypoglycemia Questionnaire" on page 184 to see if you may be suffering from hypoglycemia. If so, her treatment regimen is a good basic one to start with. Of course, self-diagnosis is just that. These are guidelines, and if you feel you are out of balance, your health practitioner should be consulted for individualized help.

### Proteins

Proteins are contained in foods such as meat, fish, and eggs, and are the building blocks of all bodily components, from hair and muscles to enzymes and hormones. Excessive protein intake encourages fat storage and can also lead to ketosis, in which muscle tissue is broken down to produce glucose for the brain. Excess protein may also contribute to osteoporosis, kidney disease, and heart disease. Proteins supply the precursors to neurotransmitters that stimulate the brain, thereby increasing alertness. So, it's a good idea to start the day with a protein-based breakfast.

### Fats

Most people don't recognize that certain fats are vital to health. The popularity of very low- to no-fat diets in recent years has actually contributed to a whole host of problems, from premenstrual syndrome (PMS) and infertility to anxiety, depression, and Attention Deficit Disorder. On the other hand, the trans-fatty acids, such as margarine and partially hydrogenated oils, cause free radical formation.

# Guidelines for a Healthy Diet

- Eat lots of fresh, organic fruits and vegetables. They provide vitamins, minerals, antioxidants, and other substances that protect against degenerative disease. They also provide necessary fiber. Whenever possible, use organic produce, since we are already overloaded with environmental toxins, and don't need more in the form of pesticides.

- Avoid processed foods. Not only are they devoid of nutritional value, they often contain dangerous additives.

- Eliminate white flour and sugar and other high-glycemic, empty-calorie foods that cause weight gain and hypoglycemia.

- Eat whole grains, which still contain their natural nutrients.

- Reduce your overall fat intake. Avoid saturated fats and fried food. Instead, eat foods rich in essential fatty acids, such as flax seed, soy, pumpkin, and walnut oils, and cold-water fish such as salmon and mackerel.

- Avoid red meat, which is high in saturated fats and contains antibiotics as well as hormones injected into the animal to fatten it. For a better source of protein, substitute skinless chicken and fish.

- Avoid soft drinks. Not only do the aluminum cans leach this toxic metal into the drink, but the drink's phosphorus content upsets electrolyte balance. The sugar in regular soft drinks is unhealthy, as is the artificial sweetener *aspartame,* a known neurotoxin. I have seen patients whose severe anxiety and even bizarre behavior cleared up when they stopped drinking aspartame-containing diet soft drinks.

- Avoid sources of caffeine, such as coffee, tea, and cola drinks.

- Limit alcohol consumption to one drink (four ounces of wine) per day.

- Drink at least eight glasses of pure water a day. Considering that our bodies are 65% water, we must not ignore this life-giving element. Many health problems will respond to adequate amounts of water.

Chlorinated tap water is not entirely healthy for you, nor are some other added minerals such as fluorine or copper. Filtered water may be preferable. However, filtered water is also lower in trace minerals, so these would need to be supplemented.

# Smoking, Alcohol Consumption, and Caffeine

## *Smoking*

Heart disease, cancer, and stroke are the three big killers in industrialized nations, and smoking is implicated in all of them. The body uses much of its available supply of vitamin C to detoxify the byproducts of smoking, leading to a vitamin C deficiency. This can result in depression, apathy, weakness, and lowered immunity.

Nicotine is a highly addictive stimulant, and withdrawal can be difficult. I have heard the accompanying tension and irritability described as "jumping out of my skin." As with the benzodiazepines, a combination of kava and valerian is useful in reducing the withdrawal symptoms. It is also easier when done in the context of a positive lifestyle change, including a good diet and nutrient program to help detoxify and rebalance your body. In addition, there is an ever-widening range of smoking cessation aids, from chewing gums, pills, and patches to books, tapes, and hypnosis. An excellent protocol for smoking cessation has been developed by therapist and EMDR practitioner A. J. Popky in Palo Alto (see Chapter 4).

## Alcohol Consumption

Alcohol consumption can cause mood swings in a process similar to hypoglycemia. It is absorbed into the bloodstream directly from the stomach without passing through the intestines. As a result, blood-sugar levels rise quickly, creating a type of sugar "high" that is part of alcohol's intoxicating effect. However, blood-sugar levels then drop, triggering a renewed desire for more alcohol or other simple sugars in order to restore blood-sugar levels. Unfortunately, such wide fluctuations ultimately contribute to a variety of mental and emotional problems, including depression.

The hypoglycemia diet and supplement program is particularly useful in dealing with the symptoms of withdrawal. These nutrients, with the addition of the amino acid glutamine, can help reduce the desire to drink. I recommend 500 to 1,000 mg twice daily, and/or whenever a craving strikes. One man with a long history of alcoholism took my advice. Simply using glutamine, he was able to stop drinking entirely, while his identical twin brother continued to drink heavily. Also, be sure to take high doses of the B vitamins and magnesium, both of which are depleted by alcohol, and vitamin C and other antioxidants for detoxification. The herb milk thistle is also good for restoring liver function, which is compromised by excessive alcohol intake. Lastly, seek help. Alcoholics Anonymous is one of a number of excellent organizations that can assist you in fighting your addiction. By the way, the heavy smoking and coffee drinking at some AA meetings is not a healthy substitute. It is often better to handle all your addictions at once, if you can.

### Caffeine Consumption

Many people say they cannot get started in the morning without that first cup of coffee. Then there are the caffeinated soft drinks and over-the-counter diet and "stay-awake" pills. Caffeine acts as a stimulant, enhancing short-term energy levels and increasing alertness. Like other stimulants, caffeine is addictive, and is often a major unrecognized component of chronic anxiety. Habitual caffeine consumption frequently leads to a syndrome known as caffeinism, which can produce anxiety and panic disorders. Other symptoms include depression, irritability, nervousness, insomnia, recurrent headaches, and heart palpitations. Many patients who complain of anxiety and insomnia are, in fact, reacting to their caffeine addiction! Another problem buried in here is the use of *aspartame,* the artificial sweetener used in soft drinks or added to coffee, which in itself can cause these same symptoms.

My advice is to avoid aspartame and caffeine altogether, or substitute Japanese green tea, in moderation. While it has some caffeine in it, it is also a good immune enhancer. My coffee-craving patients are often hypoglycemic, low adrenal ("burnout syndrome"), and hypothyroid. The solution is improved diet, exercise, and specific supplements. As you reduce your body's dependence on caffeine, you will likely find an appreciable increase in your energy level.

# Conclusion

Eat your greens, take your vitamins, and drink kava, not coffee.

In the next chapter, we will look once more at the stresses of daily life, and add tools, such as breathing and meditation, to evoke an overall sense of self awareness and mindfulness.

For more detailed dietary information, see Appendix B.

## CHAPTER 14

# Managing Stress

Life is trouble. Only death is no trouble.

*—Zorba the Greek*

The process discussed in this chapter allows a shift from our habitual reaction to stress to a more aware, present response. This state emerges more deliberate choices that include setting priorities and boundaries, as well as appropriate self-care.

## The American Dream?

I am sure that 20 years ago, none of us would have predicted our lives would look like this. Consider the following statistics.

- According to a major new study from the Families and Work Institute, Americans are working longer, harder, and faster than 20 years ago

- The time spent working each week has increased 3.5 hours in 20 years for those working 20 hours or more each week—from 43.6 hours in 1977 to 47.1 hours in 1997

- The amount of employees that say their jobs require them to work very hard is 88%—up from 70% in 1977. And 68% report having to work very fast—a 13% increase in 20 years[1]

Hours at work are cutting deeply into family time, leisure time, and just the time it takes to take care of the business of living—like shopping, cooking, or taking the dog to the vet. Compared to our pre-industrial ancestors, modern Americans spend a far larger portion of our waking hours engaged in work-related activities. An interesting paradox is that new technologies like cellular phones, faxes, and Internet-linked home computers erode our already shrunken zone of leisure time even further.

## Is There a Way Out?

A November 1996 survey by The Polling Company asked, "How willing are you to give up pay at work in exchange for more personal time?" The survey found that more than half of the respondents—55%—were willing.[2]

Many are deciding to scale back their careers or even quit lucrative jobs to spend more time with their families, some moving to smaller, less urban communities in the process. Most of us, however, can't drop out. Even if we did, our workaholic patterns might just follow us wherever we went. The answer is not *where* we play the game as much as *how* we play it.

# Getting Our Attention

Our busy, stressed, stretched lifestyles need to have some built-in ways to regroup and recharge ourselves, or we will literally wear ourselves out. Unfortunately, it is often a tragic wake-up call, in the form of a serious accident or life-threatening illness that slows us down.

## A Stressed-Out Case Study

Take, for example, Bill, a 45-year-old accountant, who went to work one morning during tax season, his busiest time, and collapsed at his desk. He luckily survived this first, serious heart attack (many don't), and was clear that things were going to change. No amount of work or responsibility was worth his life! During his hospital stay, Bill had plenty of time to think about his choices. Also, as a participant in the cardiac rehabilitation service at the hospital, he began to take a class in journal-writing. He felt like he was meeting a long-lost friend as he reconnected with forgotten parts of himself, those Inner Voices we talked about—and to—in Chapter 4.

Bill's life changed, almost by itself. As he shifted his point of view, certain activities, like working overtime, just fell away, while others, like taking walks in the nearby woods, took their place. "Where have I been?" he wondered aloud to his wife of many years. "I didn't know how much we had drifted apart, till I came back to those old feelings we had for each other in our 20s." They took the time and expense to go on a second honeymoon. Life had changed indeed.

We can blindly ignore the preciousness of life; the peace, beauty, and love that is ours. Must it take a catastrophe to wake us up? Often it does, since we human beings are creatures of habit. We need and depend on patterns of behavior. Without them, we would have to learn anew each day how to hold a fork, ride a bike, or make a phone call. On the other hand, these habits can work against us, dulling our senses and our spontaneity, turning us into robots. Unlike the child, who lives in constant wonder at the newness of life, we accommodate and adapt. When life becomes increasingly stressful, as it did for Bill, we just keep adapting—until something gives, in this case his overworked, underloving heart.

Have you heard the story of the frogs in the pot of hot water? Another case of animal experimentation, but we can still get the lesson. When frogs are placed in hot water, they jump right out. If, however, they are placed in a pot of cold water over a burner, and the heat is turned up slowly, a few degrees at a time, they remain in the pot and boil to death. This is not a recipe for frog soup. Rather, there is a moral to this story: If we are suddenly placed in a thoroughly untenable situation, like the boiling water, we recoil and escape. If, on the other hand, the situation worsens gradually, by degree, we may continue to adapt until it's too late to escape. As we lose true awareness of our surroundings and of our own feelings, the survival value of adaptation becomes a detriment.

Are you able to tell when the heat is on? Do you know how much is too much? Or have you "successfully" adapted to a self-destructive life style? Too many of us are in the latter category. What can we do to regain conscious awareness of our surroundings, to avoid becoming frog soup?

## Awareness and Self-Awareness

We have many ways of reconnecting to our inner and outer selves. We must only stay still long enough to allow it to happen. That is the paradox of awareness. Try, for example, to concentrate fully on your breathing or the chanting of a mantra. Like a two-year-old child who wants Mommy's attention, your mind will do everything it can to take your attention away from this focus. Meditation teachers call it "monkey mind," leaping from tree to tree, never still. So, total peace and quiet eludes us, even in our own minds, even on the most remote mountaintop. Is this good news or bad news?

In the words of author and mindfulness teacher Jon Kabat-Zinn, "Wherever you go, there you are." If that's the bad news, it's also the good news. What better place to start finding peace than right in your own mind? The practice of inner awareness becomes a rehearsal of your responses to the real world, in a mode of allowing surrender. As Kabat-Zinn says, "Letting go means just what it says. It's an invitation to cease clinging to anything—whether it be an idea, a thing, an event, a particular time, or view, or desire. It is a conscious decision to release with full acceptance into the stream of present moments as they are unfolding. To let go means to give up coercing, resisting, or struggling, in exchange for something more powerful and wholesome which comes out of allowing things to be as they are."[3]

Watching your breath as it goes in and out is an excellent starting place for this practice of letting go. As you allow your body to "breathe itself," interesting things start to happen. Gradually, the "out there" becomes "in here" and the "in here" becomes "out there." "I" becomes "we," and "we" become "one" as boundaries fade and disappear. For a moment, we slip into that space between the worlds. We have shifted from human "doing" to human "being."

### Practical Applications

Even done briefly, this awareness exercise is amazingly refreshing, revitalizing, and awakening in more ways than one. Our habitual patterns become clearer, and we start to see choices in our perceptions and responses. Reality is not what it used to be! We begin to notice that maybe the boss didn't mean to be critical, he was just having a rough day. Or the attractive guy or woman in the next office *is* smiling at you and meaning it, and not just being polite as you had previously thought. By slowing down, you have practiced a sharpening of your inner and outer perceptions, with better understanding of yourself and those around you. Your intuition may be sharper. You may even find yourself saying "no" to an unwanted assignment, and not even feel guilty about it.

# Our Response to Stress

As we saw earlier, stress is not simply an external factor, but a relationship between the stressor and the stressed. The result of your stress is how you respond to the provocation "out there." The more attuned you are to yourself, the better your ability to handle the normal, and sometimes excessive, stresses of life.

## *Nature, Music, and the Senses*

I was driving down the Pacific Coast Highway not long ago, or rather, I was stopped along it. Because of the winter rains, mudslides would unpredictably hold up traffic on this already narrow road, even on sunny days like this one. I was on my way to a meeting, rushing as usual, and traffic was at a dead stop. I stared at the truck in front of me, unable to see if any cars were moving up ahead. The radio report on road conditions was reduced to static, another Pacific Coast Highway peculiarity.

My jaw tightened, and my breath became shallow. I felt trapped. I looked around for an escape route and my gaze was stopped by the view out my side window. The Pacific Ocean was a sparkling blue-green, a phenomenon of California after a rain. The golden beach sand stretched down from the road to meet the white, crashing waves, and the bright blue sky was painted with fluffy, white clouds. "What am I doing to myself?" I wondered. Here, in one of the most beautiful spots I could imagine, I was complaining about being stuck in traffic! I heard the phrase "I'll get there when I get there" from somewhere inside me. I turned on a Steven Halpern tape—from his *Anti-Frantic* series. As I drank in the soothing, enlivening sound and magnificent sight, I could feel my jaw release and my breathing deepen. I was home, inside me—and outside, too. How could I have forgotten?

In a delayed reaction, I was able to voluntarily modify my response to an external stressor, the unmoving traffic, and my internal pressure to get where I was going. Nature helped me, as did the music. By the time traffic picked up again, I was fine, even sorry to leave the beautiful scene behind. Was I still late? Yes, but it just didn't seem as important. We can create and undo our own responses to stress. In a bank line, while cramming for a final, or while responding to your cranky three-year-old, take a deep breath, let go, and come back to yourself. This gives you the resources you need to handle the situation.

Music has always been a great healer. We have all heard the saying "music has charms to soothe the savage breast." In the Bible, we learn about how King Saul had his protégée, the young David, play the harp for him to help ease his severe depression. According to author and New Age music pioneer Steven Halpern, music is a significant mood-changer and de-stresser, working on many levels at once. His music plays in my waiting room, helping people to transition from their day's responsibilities and begin to focus on themselves and their needs.

I find nature to be one of the best soothers of stress. Taking a quiet walk in a park or watching a beautiful sunset can do wonders. Even reminiscing about such a scene from your past, or simply imagining one, allows your stress level to drop. Picture a trip to a palm-studded beach in Hawaii,

## Stress Control

Some people are more stress resistant than others. We might admire people who seem to thrive on chaos and perform brilliantly under pressure. What is their secret? Experts suggest that a significant determining factor between coping and burnout is your perception of the threat, as we discussed earlier. You can either worry endlessly, or you can learn to distinguish between what you can change and what is beyond your control. Research indicates that we may be able to reduce the amount of trauma caused by stress simply by determining our personal level of responsibility for events.

A few principles worth remembering:

- Life is stressful
- We determine the quality of our lives by our responses to what we encounter
- We are interdependent, and life takes place in relationships
- Don't take things personally
- Give and you will receive
- Growth involves change
- To reach our goals, we must leave our comfort zones, which usually means experiencing stress

whether you've been there or not. Or imagine a lush waterfall in Vanuatu, along with a shell of kava, of course.

### Being in the Present

As we saw in Chapter 3, past events can continue to live on inside us, causing ongoing anxiety and even insomnia. We know that while past events cannot be changed, we can

- Learn to set priorities
- Learn to say "no"
- Learn to set boundaries—and responsibilities—on time
- Some of the most popular thieves of time are interruptions, procrastination, shifting priorities, and poor planning
- Learn to be clear about what you can change and control, and what you cannot
- Life is a learning program—look for lessons
- Try not to learn the same lessons over and over again

Because we are creatures of habit and pattern, we must do the following to confront patterns:

- Learn to become aware of them
- Take responsibility for them and for confronting and changing them
- Make choices—don't be passive or act like a victim
- Don't let life happen to you
- Cultivate flexibility—in biology, it is often the key to survival

change our minds about them. The key to moving on is forgiveness—of self and others. Although it is a waste of energy to worry about future events over which we have no control, it is human nature to do so. Plan and prioritize as best you can, and then be easy on yourself. The future hasn't happened, and the past is not going to happen again. In the words of Ram Dass, "Be here now." You can start by recognizing and accepting when a situation is beyond your control.

And keep on practicing. Pythagoras said, "Choose always the way that seems the best, however rough it may be. Custom will soon render it easy and agreeable." Just as patterns and habits can trap us when we let them, we can make them our well-worn path to happiness and satisfaction.

The "Serenity Prayer" of theologian Rheinhold Niebuhr, adopted by Alcoholics Anonymous, reflects this so well:

"God grant me the serenity to accept the things I cannot change; courage to change the things I can; and the wisdom to know the difference—living one day at a time; enjoying one moment at a time; accepting hardships as the pathway to peace."

Another important sense is the sense of humor. In breathing new life into the old wisdom that "laughter is the best medicine," the late Norman Cousins transformed his own experiences into a message of healing and hope for millions.

### Exercise: Stress Relief and Much More

Stress and anxiety seem to disappear during physical activity. Most people are aware of the physical benefits of exercise: heart-lung conditioning, weight control, and bone and joint strengthening. But exercise also improves mood by producing positive biochemical changes in the body and brain. Regular exercise reduces the amount of adrenal hormones your body releases in response to stress. Also, with exercise, your body releases greater amounts of endorphins, the powerful, pain-relieving, mood-elevating chemicals in the brain. These produce the euphoric "runner's high," and also promote deep, restful sleep.

### Breathing Your Way to Relaxation

Breathing exercises are the simplest path to inner calm. Fifteen minutes a day can achieve a significant reduction in your stress-related symptoms. Breathing is one function that is controlled by both the voluntary and involuntary nervous system, forming a bridge between our inner and outer selves. There are a number of relaxation techniques that focus on breath control. One, a good sleep inducer, involves focusing on the area below the navel. Sit quietly, watching the breath as it goes in and out of your abdomen. Do this for five to ten minutes. Breath is the most natural object of meditation and an easier focus for attention than thought. If you find yourself having disturbing thoughts, instead of trying to stop them, try to simply move your attention back to your breath.

The Progressive Relaxation exercise is particularly good at bedtime. Lie down and take several deep breaths. Then breathe in slowly as you tense the muscles in your feet. Hold your breath and the tension for a count of 20. (You may not make it to 20 at the beginning.) Then, slowly breathe out, releasing the muscles until they are totally relaxed. Repeat the process with your calf muscles, and work your way up, finishing with your facial muscles. Close with a few more deep breaths. Unless, of course, you are already asleep.

### *Meditation, Biofeedback, and Neurofeedback*

Meditation, biofeedback, and neurofeedback are all powerful techniques for training the mind to distinguish between false alarms and signals of true danger. More directed in their approach than conventional psychotherapy, they tame the restless mind, helping you to deal with stress, anxiety, and insomnia. They help to promote relaxation and balance on all levels—mental, emotional, physical, and spiritual—which is the starting point for all healing. These techniques are beyond the scope of this book, but resources are provided in Appendix B for further information.

### *Attitude, Gratitude, and Service*

Optimism and a positive attitude go a long way toward maintaining good health. Research shows that the higher one's optimism, the healthier one's immune system, and

## Some Basic Tips for Stress Reduction

- Plan ahead.

- Make a to-do list in order of priorities.

- Do not bite off more than you can chew. Don't try to pack more into your day than you can cope with comfortably.

- Just say "no" to unrealistic deadlines. There is no need to feel guilty if you have to change plans or arrangements because of an impossibly tight schedule.

- Finish the most important task before you tackle the next one.

- Take regular breaks. Short rests between periods of concentrated mental effort, particularly when you are frustrated with a project or are unable to move forward, can be refreshing and help you to refocus. Five minutes of each hour or 15 minutes every two hours allows a more manageable pace.

- Take regular vacations.

- Identify the sources of your stress. This gives you more choice in how you react. If necessary, make a note of the circumstances, and see if a pattern emerges. As you delve deeper, you are more likely to discover the root of your problem, allowing you to solve it at the deepest, most effective level.

- Maintain a sense of humor about it all.

- Remember, on their deathbed, no one says, "I wish I'd spent more time at the office."

the more likely it is that good things will actually happen. Negative expectations, on the other hand, actually breed negative experiences. How do you incorporate these ideas and practices into your own life? You can begin by being grateful. No matter how bad things might appear, there is always someone who has worse problems. In fact, reaching out to such people may help you at least as much as it helps them. I have referred grieving widows and widowers, cancer survivors, and chronic fatigue patients to support groups of similar people, where they can use their experiences to help others, and be helped in the process.

## *Spiritual Needs*

Your feelings of stress or anxiety may be your mind's way of telling you to attend to your spiritual needs. The inspiration gained from spirituality is an essential part of the healing process. Mind, body, and spirit are inseparable. Making an overt connection with your spirit will provide healing for your mind and body. Prayer is a powerful healer as well. Dr. Larry Dossey's remarkable research in this area has actually proven the power of prayer. And prayer for someone else is more effective than for yourself!

Besides the organized religious groups—churches, synagogues, temples, or mosques—there are also numerous spiritual groups in which one can participate. Many offer classes and workshops. The goal in all is usually the same— to connect with the spirit, both within and without.

In the next chapter, we will look at how kava may be used to still the chatter of our inner and outer worlds, in order to help us connect with our inner selves, our communities, and with the spirit.

## CHAPTER 15

# Listening to Kava: The High Road from Doing to Being

Be still and know that I am God.

*—Psalms 46:10*

In the point of rest at the center of our being,
we encounter a world where all things are at rest in the same way.
Then a tree becomes a mystery, a cloud a revelation . . .
The life of simplicity is simple, but it opens to us a book
in which we never get beyond the first syllable.

*—Dag Hammarskjold,* Markings

## Messages of Kava

In its traditional island context, there are two essential messages of the kava experience. First, the experience is one of

peace, relaxation, ease, and well-being—even euphoria. Second, the context is social—often with a sense of ritual or ceremony.

These two qualities—well-being without tension, enjoyed in a social context—create the ideal conditions for conflict resolution. Early in this chapter we will show you how kava's traditional use for this purpose has been successfully introduced to the West. And we will briefly consider another social dimension—the relationship of kava to sex.

Then we will ask the question: What more can we learn from kava? Beyond pills for anxiety, or tinctures for tension, beyond conflict resolution—what else can it teach us? Kava has been at the core of island life for centuries, but certainly not as a treatment for anxiety. The island culture is one of kava, not of stress.

If we handle our immediate symptoms of anxiety, tension, and insomnia with kava and other herbs; if we take to heart the stress reduction lifestyle; if we even begin to break free from society's treadmill, would we still have any use for kava in our lives? What about peace of mind? What about pleasure?

What if we drink kava for the same reasons as the islanders: for inducing and sharing an experience of heightened awareness and empathy, of enhanced being, and freedom from doing? Would that be considered "getting high"? Is that recreational use? And if so, is it good or bad, moral or immoral, healthy or unhealthy? Finally, we will ask if it is worthwhile and valuable.

## Kava in Context

As we have noted in earlier chapters, kava is a deeply social beverage, both as a ritual accompaniment to celebrations, negotiations, and other occasions, and as an evening drink in the company of one's friends. The thought of a West-

erner sitting alone in a room drinking or otherwise ingest-
ing kava would strike most Pacific Islanders as strange behavior. In fact, in Fiji, the phrase "drinking kava alone" is a
euphemistic way of accusing a person of practicing black
magic.

Long used as a sacrament of welcome, kava's euphoric
qualities are best shared with special guests or friends. Kava
seems to affect the "feeling" centers where warm emotions
are generated toward those involved in the ritual.[1]

As a society, we may never reap the full benefits of this
healing herb if we continue to push ourselves beyond our
capacities for stress, tension, and conflict then, as isolated
individuals, pop a kava pill to relax. There are emotional
and physical costs to both our stress and our isolation. Having enjoyed kava in a relaxed social setting on several occasions (more about this later in the chapter), we hope to see
more social use of kava in America.

## Conflict Resolution

This link between kava and sociability isn't mere cultural
coincidence. Universally, kava users have reported that the
herb makes them feel more amiable and closer to other
human beings. Taking a cue from Pacific traditions, a growing number of doctors, herbalists, and counselors are busy
developing social uses for kava in American and European
contexts.

"Our counseling department is using kava during arbi-
trations, especially in family counseling," explains Terry
Willard, who looks like a modern-day Buddha with a beard.
He compares work at his clinics with the tradition in Fiji,
where arguing parties "sit together in a circle, share shells of
kava, calm down, settle their disputes, and life goes on. In
fact, those who were about to fight would drink the tremendously potent and ironically named 'war kava' as a stimulant

to negotiations. In this way, they were often able to resolve conflicts just before they spiraled into all-out violence."

Ever-attuned to new and innovative ways in which kava might be used, Gary Friedman tells of an experimental project in Australia using kava in the treatment of violent prison inmates. "That fits very well with how kava's used in the Pacific cultures," says Friedman, who, in addition to his kava import business, works as a chaplain to prison inmates, and is passionate about discovering new methods to help break the cycle of violence in which they find themselves trapped.

In 1937, as the world edged toward the brink of World War II, Tom Harrisson, in his book *Savage Civilization,* suggested that kava would do wonders for political and diplomatic disputes among Western nations: "It would change the face of Geneva."[2] Professor William Aalbersberg of the University of the South Pacific in Fiji puts it a bit more lightly "Pacific meetings don't end until all agree. Of course, using kava makes it easier. Those who don't agree, fall asleep."

In my own practice, I have found kava particularly effective in helping individuals handle disputes.

### Kava Helps Resolve Disputes

Take, for example, the case of Tony and Dan, two men in their late 20s. They had started a construction business together several years earlier, but their respective plans changed, and their lives began to move in different directions. Dan, still single, wanted to expand the business rapidly, while Tony, married and a father, wished to stabilize operations and spend more time with his family. Both men were disappointed, angry, and worried that a tough legal battle over splitting up the company was inevitable—and bound to be costly on all levels.

They hoped to find a way to ease the inevitable breakup of the partnership while still preserving their friendship. They decided to use a third party to help mediate the situation, and I was chosen. My approach was to set up a meeting, preceded by the two men taking a mild dose of kava—

250 mg of 30% standardized kavalactones, in tincture form for rapid delivery. The kava helped reduce the men's anxiety and potential impulsiveness, promoting a quiet inner and social space in which to experience feelings of trust and safety. Dan described the sensation as, ". . . remarkable! I knew I was upset, but I was able to formulate my ideas and express them clearly and kindly, without the anger that I had felt before. I could even express my disappointment without blaming Tony. I'm so glad we didn't escalate and say things we would later regret."

The business still broke up, but the men dissolved the partnership without the time, expense, and heartbreak that a legal fight would have entailed. They have not only remained friends, but their communication actually improved, deepening their long-standing friendship. While this may seem surprising to most of us, to the South Sea islanders, mediation with kava is a way of life that has been successful for hundreds of years.

I have likewise used it to ease communication in couples' counseling with equally positive results.

---

## Kava and Sex

Some of the initial interest in kava in the United States and Europe focused on another social use: To capitalize on rumors that the herb is a sexual stimulant, products appeared on the shelves with names like "Erotikava" and "Kava Sutra." So, does it work? Although research still needs to be conducted in the area, anecdotal evidence suggests that by relaxing the body, particularly the pelvic region, kava does seem to work as an aphrodisiac for women.

In addition, kava breaks down barriers, enhances communication, and produces a feeling of contentment, all of which can promote and enhance intimate encounters. In our culture, this role is often filled by alcohol or other inebriants.

Unlike alcohol, however, kava does not dull the senses. In fact, it actually enhances perception on many levels, including heightening sensual feelings.

However, according to Carleton Gajdusek, at the United States government's Ethnopharmacological Search for Psychoactive Drugs Symposium in San Francisco in 1967, "it is quite evident that kava drinkers rarely engage in sexual activity on the nights when they drink".[3] On most of the islands, until recently, women were not allowed to drink kava except medicinally. Today, however, a man likes his woman to drink kava to relax into her sensuality. But he doesn't drink it with her, because the same muscle relaxation might interfere with his performance.

## The Fresh Kava Experience

Many Westerners are reluctant to describe kava's effects in terms reminiscent of recreational drugs. Yet it remains an undeniable fact that when you take kava, at least in the manner and forms used regularly in the South Pacific, your consciousness is unmistakably altered. It's difficult to improve on the description of anthropologist E. M. Lemert, who in 1967 observed, "The head is affected pleasantly; you feel friendly, not beer sentimental. Kava quiets the mind; the world gains no new color or rose tint; it fits in its place and in one easily understandable whole."[4] Referring to its subtlety, islanders say: "Kava doesn't come to you. You go to kava."

Contemporary Westerners who drank the beverage made from powder, as opposed to tinctured extracts or pills, describe their experiences in similar terms. Witness the following two quotes from kava users: "I was seriously relaxed in a pleasant sort of way, but I didn't seem to be incapacitated at all. I went into the kava in a very lousy mood. I was tired, mentally overdrawn, and generally in a sort of disgruntled humor—or worse. After it kicked in though, I was relaxed. I was still aware of all of the deadlines and such hovering over me, but they all seemed to be put in perspective." The other user reports, "For me anyway, it's worth the super unpleasant taste to get the effect. One's mind is not fogged, but the spirit is at rest; very relaxed. It also seems to act as a muscle relaxant. At higher doses, one may be inclined to lay down and not move a muscle. It's definitely something to do in the evening, several hours before bedtime. Sleepiness occurs after about an hour. Kava also gives me great and very vivid dreams coupled with an extremely restful, deep sleep."

# Drugs: Hard and Soft

Imagine people openly claiming serious relaxation after drinking kava for pleasure. American society has a strangely bifurcated view toward people using chemicals to alter their mind states. On the one hand, potent "psychotropic" or mood altering drugs such as Prozac, Valium, and Xanax are prescribed so frequently that we seem on our way to Aldous Huxley's *Brave New World* vision of a chemically pacified society. Yet, for most of American history, the use of drugs for anything other than medical therapeutic purposes has been treated as a threat to society. With a few state-sanctioned exceptions, such as caffeine, alcohol, and nicotine, chemicals used for purposes of recreation, pleasure, or insight are strictly prohibited. Their users are punished and incarcerated in an ever-more draconian and unsuccessful "war on drugs."

We agree that much drug taking is negative and destructive to individuals, families, and communities. But this hardly applies to the pursuit of enhanced presence, awareness, or empathy through drinking kava. We are not defending hard drugs such as heroin or cocaine, which are unlikely to lead to enlightenment, but we suggest openness to substances that may be capable of expanding consciousness in a positive way—kava among them.

As Nathan Kline of Rockland State Hospital, Orange-burg, New York, expressed at the Ethnopharmacological Conference of 1967, "Pharmaceuticals, like firearms, in themselves can be described only by such terms as potent or precise. Not their effectiveness, but their application, determines whether they are 'good' or 'bad'."[5]

## Some Background Information

The conference mentioned above, sponsored by the National Institute of Mental Health in 1967 in San Francisco, explored an array of psychoactive plants from around the world. Kava was a primary focus, and the proceedings became a major source of information, providing some of the material for this book. It attracted a "who's who" of people in the field of psychiatry and ethnopharmacology, including Daniel X. Freedman, later president of the American Psychiatric Association; Richard Schultes, renowned Harvard ethnobotanist; Nathan Kline, then at Rockland State Hospital; Gordon Wasson of Harvard University; Carl Pfeiffer, a leader in orthomolecular medicine; Claudio Naranjo, famed Chilean psychiatrist and author; Alexander Shulgin, author and innovative pharmacologist at the University of California, San School, and Andrew Weil, now an influential spokesperson for integrative medicine. Perhaps we are seeing a reawakening of interest in psychoactive plants. For example, the esteemed British medical journal *Lancet* recently published a positive review of *TIKHAL,* Shulgin's latest book on the subject.

## Responsible Use

Both marijuana and kava promote a sense of relaxation and camaraderie. Unlike marijuana, however, when used in moderation, kava has no dulling effect on perception or mental dexterity. As mentioned in Chapter 11, a placebo-controlled research study that tested driving skills actually showed enhancement of these skills in the kava group compared to the placebo group.[6] This is not to say that an excessive dose will not diminish driving skills. Good judgment must always be used when taking a mind- and mood-altering substance.

# Roots of Consciousness

It may be safe to say that early plants, dating back over three billion years, provided the foundation for the development of all subsequent forms of plants and, later, of animals, including that most recent of creatures, the human being. It remains one of the unsolved riddles of nature why certain plants produce substances with specific effects on the mind and emotions of man, on his sense of perception, and actually on his state of consciousness. In nonindustrial societies, plants that alter the mind and body have always been considered sacred.

The use of substances to alter consciousness has been part of human life throughout history and in every corner of the globe. We have had an urge to transcend our limits, to escape reality, or to relieve anxiety. We do so through magic, drama, ritual, physical extremes, dreams, and drugs. UCLA researcher Dr. Ron Siegel speaks for others working in the field when he claims, "There is a natural force that motivates the pursuit of intoxication." In fact, the brains of humans and animals produce specific chemicals in response to pleasurable experiences, and the same receptors that receive these internally produced messages seem to be the ones that respond to external stimuli as well. There are biofeedback techniques and devices that help train the brain to release its own endorphins and other neurochemicals to create a natural high. In the greater scheme of things, a person using kava to relax isn't so different from one who feels pleasure from watching the sunset, laughing at a friend's joke, or enjoying a good massage.

Finally, if as Andrew Weil suggests in his book *The Natural Mind,* "the desire to alter consciousness periodically is an innate drive analogous to hunger or the sexual drive," kava seems to be one of the safest, least addictive mind-altering substances currently available.[7] Dr. Weil is a current proponent of kava's use in treating anxiety.

## Experiencing Kava

We have had the good fortune on several occasions of enjoying fresh kava in a social setting. The roots have an energy about them. Growers treat them with much respect and pride. They offer each other their prize cultivars, then watch expectantly for drinkers' reactions. But it doesn't feel competitive because they are all drinking kava. To paraphrase the island saying, "you can't compete with kava in you."

There is a subtle, but knowing, excitement in the room when the kava comes out. Folks are eager to drink and to enter into the kava energy, which begins to connect the people in the room. With all this awareness of the group experience, kava's effects are quite internal, as well. The quicker the tongue goes numb, the stronger the kava. The taste is always potent. It grabs the inside of my mouth. But I don't mind. I find it has a wonderful aftertaste that lingers.

Over the next several minutes, at least four things seem to happen fairly simultaneously. A wave of relaxation rolls through my body. We have said throughout the book that the effects of kava are immediate; immediate, but not abrupt. Kava happens to me. My body is very alive and aware, but free of tension. The second thing that happens is an emotional release, perhaps even more subtle than the physical. I don't notice the change as it happens, but I find

I'm feeling at ease, comfortable in my skin, but again, very awake. Vision and hearing are slightly heightened. I've read of the islanders' wanting silence and darkness because of increased sensitivity, but I've never found it uncomfortable. Both sights and sounds are just a little brighter, clearer, and warmer.

Finally I'm aware of a feeling of easy connectedness and relationship with others in the room. Some I know well, others I've never met before. Mentally I note a couple of people whose personalities might normally push my buttons. But not tonight. I walk around and observe groups of two and three in animated conversation. Alert and at ease, people focus on each other, paying close attention. My own conversations are thoroughly engaging, with a flow that feels solid. In the course of the next couple of hours, no one argues, no one yells, no one seems out of place. There is a sense of belonging and of genuine interest in each other. People want to be truly seen and heard in life, and tonight it feels to me as if they are. After maybe three drinks of kava, it's after 11:00 P.M. and I'm beginning to lose steam. I offer goodbyes and a few heartfelt hugs and head out.

When islanders speak of "listening to kava," they refer to the naturally contemplative awareness it brings. I listen that way, but I also listen for kava's bigger message. Kava is quiet, internal, and social. Kava is about presence and being in the moment. It seems to open a window to subtle knowledge and awareness, and connection to nature as well as to others and to oneself.

## Kava Ultimately Relieves Stress

Finally, let us compare the qualities of the stressful environment we repeatedly confront in our daily lives to the qualities of kava.

| Stressful Environment | Kava |
|---|---|
| sleep deprivation | REM sleep, renewal |
| stress | rest, relaxation |
| anxiety | calm |
| speed | rhythm |
| noise | quiet |
| tension | release |
| rigidity | flow |
| competition | cooperation, sharing |
| physical contraction | breathing |
| fear | trust |
| hostility | well-being, empathy |
| danger | safety |

The kava experience and the kava culture present a set of qualities we desperately need to cultivate in our lives. Kava offers heightened awareness amid peace and well-being; conditions highly favorable for health as well as for growth.

In the next chapter, we will look at the agriculture of kava in various islands of the Pacific and discuss questions of compensation between indigenous farmers and multinational corporations.

## CHAPTER 16

# Growing Kava

Throughout this book, we have shown how kava has a valuable role to play in helping to cope with stress and anxiety by providing physical, emotional, and mental relaxation naturally and without side effects. In sum, kava can help us achieve healthier, more productive, more balanced lives.

In the next two chapters, we are going to investigate several aspects of the world of kava that may determine the scope of its impact. We have said all along that things exist within larger contexts. Most stress occurs in a social context. Kava grows in a natural context, and its use emerges from a cultural context. Its effects are experienced in a physical context—all interrelated systems.

There is a centuries-old tradition of herbal medicine that presents itself today within a global economic market. Kava has been cultivated for generations by families of island men, as it is today. Kava makes its way to our office drawers and our night tables through a web of relationships and exchanges between people of very different worlds.

We will look at potential problems for kava at both the supply and demand ends of the spectrum. By ignoring its cultural context, we in the United States may misuse or abuse the herb. Even its appropriate use may face economic and regulatory obstacles created by ill-informed political or cultural forces or by the self-serving power of the pharmaceutical industry. On the other hand, the timing of kava's popularity may be excellent. Society needs the relief kava has to offer. More and more people know about and prefer natural, nontoxic, nonaddicting treatments. Kava could ride several trends over the next few years to become a household word, making life more manageable and enjoyable for millions.

## Opportunities and Obstacles

The kava plant, ideally suited for both the climate and the economy of the South Pacific, continues to increase in importance as a major cash crop, for domestic use as well as for export. In the case of kava, islanders are growing a product that they still use as part of their traditional culture, unlike so many other cash crops that developing nations grow simply for export. Kava growing can contribute to sustainable development, while providing a valuable product to the world market, thereby helping post-colonial Pacific Island nations to address important issues in their struggling new economies.

There are potential obstacles to fully realizing this vision. Asesela Ravuvu, social science professor at the University of the South Pacific and a member of the Fijian President's Council, raises several social and economic challenges confronting the evolving kava industry in its native islands:

- Rural people need economic opportunities so that they can earn a living where they live, rather than having to move to urban centers

- There is a lurking threat that the kava industry will move away from the rural people who have always grown it

- Commercialization of kava cultivation must be undertaken with care

- To expand productivity of kava may call for introducing new or expanded technologies, but this must be done without harming the local environment

- The expansion of kava cultivation must not come at the cost of food production[1]

To examine these problems properly, we will begin with the traditional cultivation of kava, then move on to the significant economic factors.

There is an enormous variety of cultivars with varying chemical properties and differing above-ground appearances. Although the kava roots show little external variation (except, according to Vincent Lebot, "the yellower the roots, the better the kavalactones"), they produce an enormous range of effects when ingested.[2] The actual genetic base of kava's actions is very narrow. Out of 10,000 genes, perhaps two or three are responsible for all of kava's chemical properties. Plants grown in the same garden, planted on the same day, and picked on the same day vary greatly, though predictably. Only certain genetically determined chemotypes, with the ideal proportions of specific kavalactones, will produce particular desired effects. Although farmers may sample *all* their plants, they will propagate only those with the effects they prefer.

Kava thrives in the very rich soil of volcanic islands. Planting kava with other crops is best, although one must be careful that the other crops are not hosts for its enemies.

Intercropping between coconut, coffee, noni, macadamia nuts, or other tree crops is good, as kava does well in shade. Kava is also suitable for intercropping with food crops, such as papaya, banana, yams, and sweet potatoes. Even though kava roots should be five to seven years old before being picked, they still produce a quicker return than timber. In addition, the kava for export is often harvested sooner, since it is not grown for the subtle effects preferred by the natives. Relatively quick to mature and fairly simple to process, kava provides a high cash return for labor expended.

## Vanuatu and Fiji

Vanuatu, formerly the New Hebrides, consists of more than 80 islands spread over more than 800 kilometers, with only one commercial center, Port Vila. It is much less developed than Fiji or Samoa, with little electrical power, and few wharves. Unlike some of the other island nations, however, Vanuatu is said to retain a fairly strong system of traditional governance, through island and village chiefs.

Kava is grown in family plots connected to villages. It's best to be near a creek for washing, with good access to sun for drying. According to Vincent Lebot, rain can be a major problem in Vanuatu, producing mold that can quickly destroy seven years of growth and centuries of cultivation. Farmers have to be ready at any moment to protect the harvested roots from the rain.[3]

From kava plots scattered all over the far-flung hills, the roots are harvested, dried, put into jute sacks, and carried to collection points. Often this means carrying sacks of kava over the mountains for dozens of miles to a road or coastal spot where a boat can land. Eventually the sacks find their way to Port Vila, where they are shipped to other parts of the world.[4]

"You've got a third world country, with a very proud people who've learned the lessons of colonialism in the

Pacific," says Gary Friedman of Cosmopolitan Trading, a kava exporter. "They've seen what heavy industry, mining, excessive tourism, and the rest have done to other places. Kava is a part of their culture and their economy that can provide them a way out of the dependence on foreign aid that hurts so many developing countries. There's something wonderful in the fact that a crop they've grown and used for 3,000 years just might be their economic salvation."

Ed Smith of HerbPharm in Oregon observes, "I'm hearing stories about companies wanting to start kava plantations in places like Haiti or Mexico, where labor's really cheap and they can use lots of pesticides, and I'm sure that will happen." But, he assures me, "there will always be a demand for the really good, mature kava from places like Vanuatu, where it's been organically grown in a sustainable manner."

Vanuatu produces 8,000 tons of fresh kava for drinking per year, but the people consume so much locally that it leaves little for export. Many locals drink daily. Kava bars in town serve kava for $1 per cup, less than a beer. On a positive note, the island sends regular health reports to the World Health Organization, which so far has found no side effects in daily drinkers.[5]

With the increasing demands of commerce, Vanuatu's enthusiastic and innovative young kava farmers are advancing beyond their inherited knowledge. They have found kava can produce a 100% success rate when planted on the sides of tarrow ponds, in partnership with vines, which combat destructive nematodes. A growing concern, however, is that today's farmers are tending toward *monoculture,* cultivation of a single crop, rather than using the land for multiple purposes, and sacrificing genetic variety in the process. As a crop integrated with other crops, kava mimics nature, whereas monoculture favors pests and disease.

In Fiji, kava is more likely to be grown plantation-style, and the plantations are more likely to be controlled by East Indians, rather than native Fijians. Fiji also has greater infrastructure than Vanuatu. Due to all these factors, the kava industry in Fiji is more mature, and has long been the primary source for much of the European and American markets.

One acre of kava takes several years to produce two tons of dry root. To meet growing worldwide demand for kava extract there will need to be many, many more acres planted. "We're okay now," according to Friedman, "but things might change if kava turns into another St. John's wort in terms of public awareness and demand. After all, you can't just stick kava in the ground and harvest it the next month." Ed Smith echoes this concern, "I'm afraid we'll see some adulteration of product if kava demand outstrips supply. The temptation will be great for some companies to use the really young [and less potent] roots."

# Hawaii

If the biggest current producers in Vanuatu and Fiji have problems producing enough for increased global markets due to the lack of infrastructure and the tendency to overconsume kava locally, Hawaii is eager to fill the gap. Economic and agricultural development forces on the island see an opportunity for Hawaii, which was hit hard over the last decade by local losses in the pineapple and sugarcane industries. It was with that in mind that the state hosted The First International Botanical Symposium on Kava and Other Medicinal Plants of the South Pacific in Kona, Hawaii in 1997 which was described at the start of this book.

Hawaii has been devastated by harsh business practices. As local plantations closed, their jobs went overseas in search of cheaper labor. Hawaii Kava Growers, a network of small farmers, was formed to share knowledge and experience and to assure that its members are practicing business for the good of all. The growers hope that kava can become a low-impact, sustainable agricultural product (LISA). They believe an ideal standard for the market and the industry would be that each of the participants profit in proportion to the risk they undertake. Jerry Konanui, the group's physically imposing vice president, expresses himself with a dignity born of a life of hard work in paradise. "When you harvest, you must replant. When you take, you must give back."

In ancient Hawaii, diversity was the name of the game, and the idea of monocropping didn't make sense to a society that produced all their own needs without imports. Though monoculture as practiced on the plantation was unsustainable, it produced short- and middle-term profits for big growers, and replaced a sustainable system that had worked for 1,000 or more years in Hawaii. Attempts at large plantation plantings of kava have met with failure so far, due to the usual reasons that a monoculture fails: root disease, nematodes, leaf diseases, and the appearance of new insect pests brought on by the sudden supply of a new host.

The very nature of kava cultivation through propagation of cuttings rather than planting of seeds may be better suited to individual growers and their co-ops rather than to the massive monoculture farms of agribusiness. We are likely to see the development and failure of more kava plantations. Family plots and small intercropped plantations will have the advantage. According to Robert Faust, Ph.D., if small growers successfully organize themselves in order to contend in the competitive market, kava could ultimately emerge as the best small farm crop in the traditional kava growing areas of Hawaii. The area now known as the Kona coffee belt was, prior to Western contact, the taro and 'awa' belt.

# Questions of Compensation

The coming century is already being termed "the age of biology," or *The BioTech Century*, the title of a new book by Jeremy Rifkin. Products derived from biological materials are expected to increasingly replace those made from metals

## The Gene Rush

The issues of bioengineering and the patenting of life forms present significant challenges to society's abilities to reckon with the interaction of biology, morality, and economics. Though hardly front page news in the United States, today's decisions and precedents are likely to have enormous impact in the years to come. A few examples of current developments:

- An Indian seeds company paid $2 million to a U.S. agribusiness firm for two grams of seed of a U.S. cotton variety patented by the seller, who was initially demanding $10 million.

- At the U.N. Women's Conference in Beijing, 118 indigenous groups from 27 countries signed a declaration demanding "a stop to the patenting of all life forms" which is "the ultimate commodification of life, which we hold sacred."

- In May 1995, leaders of 80 religious faiths and denominations (including the Protestant, Catholic,

and chemicals. Genes of living organisms are the basic "raw materials" of the new biotechnologies. People in developing countries are now aware of the huge profits being reaped by companies involved in what is often termed "bio-piracy" and are fighting back.

Transnational corporations are being granted patents for products and technologies that make use of the genetic materials of plants and other biological resources that have long been identified, developed, and used by farmers and indigenous peoples, mainly in countries of the south. While

Muslim, Hindu, Buddhist, and Jewish faiths) held a joint press conference in Washington announcing their opposition to the patenting of genetically engineered animals and human genes, cells, and organs.

Farmers' Rights, which recognize farmers' contributions to germplasm development and their right to share in any benefits derived from commercial or other use, were accepted by the United Nations Food and Agriculture Organization in 1985 and at the Rio Earth Summit in 1992.

While a legally binding treaty on the exchange of germplasm is being worked out, nearly half a million seed varieties from around the world are being administered under a trusteeship between crop research centers and the United Nations Food and Agriculture Organization. The challenge for those campaigning against life patents is to ensure that within the Biodiversity Convention, the World Trade Organization develops the case against bio-piracy and concrete measures to counter it.[6, 7]

corporations stand to make huge revenues from this process, the local communities often go unrewarded and face the threat in the future of having to buy the products of these companies at high prices.

As demand for kava in "advanced" countries grows, the native islanders who are responsible for its discovery, propagation, and survival face complex threats of economic exploitation and cultural dislocation. Kava growers face a situation similar to that of the indigenous peoples of the rain forests, whose medicinal plants are being harvested by pharmaceutical companies for product development. The kava industry provides an opportunity for developing sustainable economic relationships that serve the interests of all concerned.

Many South Pacific Islanders see kava as their cultural, traditional, and community property which Westerners, including Hawaiians, intend to take away from them and commercialize. They see themselves as the ones who kept kava alive through the years of its suppression by missionaries. Even now, some are torn between the ritual and community use of kava and the economic opportunities it offers. There is talk of halting the flow of seed stock and cuttings outside of Polynesia to prevent its being grown outside the region.

Although it is difficult to share Oceania's knowledge, since much of it is sacred, Dr. William Aalbersberg of the University of the South Pacific in Fiji passionately believes herbal commercial development should, at the very least, follow the Pacific way of reciprocity. South Pacific nations want to participate in the processing of their resources, not merely their growing and harvesting. He points out the potential for win-win arrangements, where lower island labor costs could benefit foreign investors, while providing jobs and income to the local communities.

# Intellectual Property
# Rights—and Wrongs

The peoples of the Pacific have developed knowledge and breeds, but they have done so communally and over time, in ways not recognized by Western concepts of intellectual property rights (IPR). Examples of protected intellectual property include trade secrets, patents, plant breeders, rights, trademarks, and copyrights. Intellectual property rights seek to:

- Provide incentives to inventors

- Promote public disclosure of technology to lead to its transfer

- Reward effort

- Satisfy the moral right

Finding current IPR systems inappropriate for the primary holders of Pacific intellectual property, advocates have devised a covenant called "Traditional Resource Rights" as a way to protect indigenous traditional knowledge. They are putting forward new ideas such as discovery rights, defensive publication, and community knowledge registers. The key provisions of the covenant on Traditional Resource Rights are as follows:

- Any use of locally developed resources or knowledge calls for upfront funding of all costs to be incurred by the community

- An independent monitor must evaluate all agreements, to ensure that all parties understand and comply

- Prior informed consent must be obtained through full disclosure

- Concern must be shown for the biological and social environment

- Benefits and profits must be shared equitably

The goals of the 1992 Convention on Biological Diversity are the conservation of biodiversity, the sustainable development of genetic resources, and fair and equitable sharing of benefits. According to its provisions, nations have sovereign rights to sustainable development of their resources; nations should provide access to genetic resources in return for technology transfer on terms mutually agreed to by both parties; and indigenous knowledge should be protected and fair benefits given for its use.

# Conclusion

In this chapter, we watched the supply of kava move from the growers to the exporters, looking at issues of cultivation and compensation. Now, we will move to the countries of the West and explore kava's marketing, distribution, and regulation.

## CHAPTER 17

# The Economics and Regulation of Kava

As we have covered nearly every other aspect of kava, now let's examine the international and American markets for herbal medicine, the regulation of plant medicines in Europe and in America, and kava's growing presence in the marketplace.

## The Herbal Medicine Market— Europe and North America

As you are aware by now, Europeans have a very different official relationship with medicinal plants than we in the United States. Herbal or natural medicine is the original traditional medicine. Approximately 500 plants are sources of contemporary medicines that result in estimated annual sales of over a $100 billion. The first European document on the properties and uses of medicinal plants, composed in the first century A.D. by the Greek physician Dioscorides, remained a major reference into the 1600s. Several European nations, including Germany, France, and Italy, have never turned their backs on what are called "phytomedicines." In these countries, the use of such medicines is recognized, regulated, and often (40% in Germany and France) reimbursed by health insurance.

In other countries, Great Britain and the Netherlands among them, the situation is similar to the United States, where herbal treatments are considered food supplements without medicinal value. The emerging European Union will change this divided picture over the next few years, until plant medicines will be treated as drugs, and registrations, based on quality, safety, and efficacy will be required. In any case, the herbal medicine market continues to grow rapidly throughout Europe.

By definition, phytomedicines are based solely on plant material, and either the complete plant or its extracts are used in treatment. In Asia, complementary and conventional medicines are practiced in parallel. The world buys $14 billion worth of herbal remedies. Europe accounts for half of that total: with Germany at 50% and France at 25%.[1] Citizens of the European community spend an average of $17.50 (United States) per year on herbal medicines, and 80% of German physicians prescribe them.[2] In Germany, St. John's wort outsells Prozac by at least five to one. Forty percent of German medicines are based on plant material.[3] In the United States, the figure is more than 20%.[4]

To put things in perspective and to visualize the enormous room for growth, sales of botanical or herbal products in the United States now exceed $3 billion, while sales of all pharmaceuticals amount to between $50 and $60 billion.[5]

According to the most recent survey, 32% of adults spend an average of $54 per year on herbal remedies for a total of $3.24 billion. Despite this, North America still lags far behind Europe in both use and research. As we have seen, most scientific papers on plant medicine are published in European journals.[6] It is also interesting that the major European suppliers of herbs are pharmaceutical companies. This is cause for some concern in the United States among more traditional herb suppliers, as it seems possible that the European pharmaceutical/herb giants may take over the market here.

# Regulation: Commission E and the FDA

Based on safety and efficacy data, Commission E of the German Federal Health Agency has published more than 230 positive monographs on herbs in the Federal Register. The European Scientific Cooperative for Phytomedicines (ESCOP) is preparing European monographs or summaries of products' characteristics (SPCs), to be used as the basis for European Union registrations.

The U.S. Food and Drug Administration (FDA), which regulates over-the-counter, herbal medications, does not readily accept research-based information from outside the United States. Unil recently, no medical claims were allowed in any case. The Dietary Supplement Health and Education Act of 1994 (DSHEA), which is described below, made an initial step in the right direction, allowing limited claims for herbs as dietary supplements. Though therapeutic or drug claims are still not allowed, changes in the structure and function of the human body by herbs can now be mentioned in advertisements and product labels.

# Growing American Interest
# in Herbal Medicine

Donald Brown, M.D., director of Natural Products Research Consultants and editor of the *Natural Products Quarterly Review,* reviewed an editorial from the respected medical journal, *The Lancet,* on the subject of herbal medicine. Content aside, there is great significance to the fact that this conservative journal is devoting space to a discussion of this topic. "This editorial points out both the enormous growth of pharmaceutical industry interest and the critical need for expanded research. Fifteen years ago none of the top 250 pharmaceutical companies had research programs involving higher plants. Today, over half of them do. However, support for plant-based research continues to be overlooked by most funding bodies. Less than 10% of the estimated quarter of a million flowering plant species in the world have been examined scientifically for their healing potential. Sixty thousand species of higher plants will probably become extinct by the year 2050. This demands a sense of urgency. Ethnobotany, the study of medicinal plants, must be an international priority."[7]

Plant extracts have proven effective in treating some chronic conditions for which conventional medicine has offered little therapeutic relief. The World Health Organization estimates that 80% of the world's population relies on plant-based medicines for primary health care. This makes it clear that there is knowledge available. It also points out the need for research and development, to test for the safety and efficacy of traditional remedies, and to standardize their effective use. It is also important that practitioners develop standardized and accurate methods of reporting their clinical findings. "Real-life" results are as important as controlled clinical studies, not only to keep alive and reinforce common uses of plant medicines, but also to continue to expand their use into new areas.

According to Mark Blumenthal and the American Botanical Council, sales of herbal supplements—which have long been found primarily in health food outlets—rose dramatically in drugstores and supermarkets in 1994. Compared to 1993, sales increased 32% in drugstores, totaling $74.7 million, and increased 41% in food stores to $31.9 million. The average growth for both outlets was 35%, totaling $106.7 million in retail sales.[8]

# Going Mainstream

---

This expansion into mainstream markets continues. In a 1998 study, Hartman and New Hope surveyed 43,442 households, tracing what products consumers use to supplement their diets. Among the findings:

- The amount of American households that consumed a vitamin, mineral, or herbal supplement in the previous six months was 68%

- The amount of those surveyed who purchased their dietary supplements at a pharmacy or drug store was 24%

- The amount that went to the grocery store for their needs was 17%.[9]

A majority of kava product marketers promote kava as a calming, relaxing, and safe dietary supplement—an alternative to Valium, Prozac, or even Sominex. They tend to soft-pedal its more exotic South Pacific cultural history. Their targeted customer is the workaholic baby boomer who wants less stress but sharper thinking during working hours; or that same person who wants to calm down in a suburban home after an hour and a half in traffic.

# Money Talks

---

Due to an aging population, direct consumer advertising of prescription products, faster approval of drugs by the Food and Drug Administration, and a willingness to substitute pharmaceuticals for other therapies, health care providers are spending more on drugs these days than ever before. In 1997, pharmaceutical company profits jumped from 15% to 20%.[10]

Financial muscle seems to go a long way toward explaining why pharmaceuticals are acceptable over natural products. For example, at about the time that Prozac was introduced, the natural antidepressant amino acid tryptophan was banned by the FDA due to adverse reactions to a single contaminated batch. Contrast this with the case of Tylenol, a highly promoted product of a major pharmaceutical corporation. Once the source of contamination was discovered, appropriate precautions taken to protect future product, and significant public relations dollars spent, it was restored to the shelves.

Tryptophan, despite being regulated as a dire health threat, continued to be found in infant formula and in parenteral feeding, i.e., high nutrient feeding for debilitated patients. Apparently, these markets weren't competing with Prozac. The FDA has historically demonstrated a harmful anti-supplement bias, though there are signs of a growing willingness to dialogue regarding their merits.

The pharmaceutical industry spends large sums of money on research because of the potential financial rewards of patentability. Since it is difficult to patent herbs, and thus more difficult to attain exclusivity in the marketplace, there is less potential financial return on research. Even much university-based research is heavily subsidized by the pharmaceutical industry, leading to potential bias in results. As we've pointed out, this is much less true in Europe, where most herbal research has been done. This is likely because the European manufacturers customarily protect their research and development with "proprietary products," something that is starting to happen more in America.

Product quality also remains a critical issue. In contrast to chemical substances, plants vary in their composition, therefore quality must be controlled carefully. The isolation and quantification of active ingredients is costly in terms of time and money. Additionally, for new medical claims the FDA is likely to demand clinical trials with price tags in the $200 to $500 million range.

Critics say that an FDA regulation regarding clinical trials, proposed in 1994 and expected to take effect soon, will greatly increase the cost of trials for new drugs. Medical researchers at the Johns Hopkins University Center for Clinical Trials carefully compared two clinical trials, one under the old reporting requirements and one under the new rules, and concluded that the FDA's changes would increase the costs of a single trial by $24 million. In 1997, Congress passed and the president signed a bill to speed up the FDA's drug approval process and reduce the cost of developing new drugs—which had increased from an average of $359 million in 1990 to $500 million in 1993.

# The FDA and DSHEA:
# Dietary Supplement Health and
# Education Act of 1994

In 1985, when some larger than usual shipments of a little known South Pacific herb showed up on a dock in Los Angeles, the Food and Drug Administration detained them, declaring that kava was an unapproved food additive. A year later, in response to requests from Fiji, the FDA decided that under certain conditions, they would allow kava in: If it was to be used only as food or drink, with a limit of 300 mg per day, and as long as no therapeutic claims were made.

In 1994, more Americans spoke to Congress about the regulation of botanical supplements than about any issue since the end of the Vietnam War. Passage of the Dietary Supplement Health and Education Act (known as DSHEA) set new guidelines with regard to quality, labeling, packaging, and marketing of supplements. It also sparked a surge of interest in herbal products, including kava.

When the FDA looks at a substance, it asks if it is a dietary supplement, an over-the-counter medicine, a prescription medicine, or a food. According to the FDA, "use determines category," so there is no traditional medicine category.[11] In dealing with the FDA, there are three options as to how herbal products can be defined and regulated. They can be considered old drugs, new drugs, or dietary supplements. The FDA has been cool about considering them old drugs, which would, in a sense, "grandfather" their approval, without calling for expensive research trials. The "new drug" qualification process is not affordable for a non-patentable herb. So most herbal products, including kava, are regulated as dietary supplements.

DSHEA allows manufacturers to make "statements of nutritional support for conventional vitamins and minerals," but since herbs aren't nutritional in the conventional sense, DSHEA allows them to make only what they call "structure and function claims." They can explain how the vitamin or herb affects the structure or function of the body. However, they can make no therapeutic or prevention claims, such as "Treats headaches fast," or "Cures the common cold."

A company can say that the herb saw palmetto helps maintain urinary and prostate health in men 50 and up. But they can't say it helps treat the symptoms associated with benign prostatic hypertrophy, which is the actual reason people use it. That would mention the pathology and the treatment, and be considered a drug claim. Companies use verbal acrobatics in labeling products, so as not to fall over this line.

This situation is far from perfect. A patient came to see me recently, wanting to take St. John's wort, but she was concerned. "My mother-in-law said that it's a dangerous MAO inhibitor and requires a special diet. I also heard that you sunburn when you take it, and that you can't take it with alcohol." These warnings were, for the most part, untrue, but with some basis in fact. There is too little guidance for people like her. If the manufacturer could include the equivalent of a German Commission E enclosure with each bottle, then people could be properly informed. They wouldn't be as confused by all of the contradictory things they hear.

At this point, the Commission E monographs are available in English (including an exhaustive collection published by the American Botanical Council), but this pertinent information cannot be enclosed in a box with an herbal product. That would be considered drug labeling. The report can be put out as what's called "third-party literature" by the herbal company, as long as they don't put the company's name on the booklet or display stand. This opportunity to distribute third-party literature is one of the best provisions of DSHEA, along with allowing a label listing adverse side effects and warnings. Prior to this, the FDA's policy had been "Foods don't have warnings, only drugs have warnings." And herbs had been considered foods.

The Commission E monographs offer a model for how to go beyond the Dietary Supplements Act and begin to develop an expert panel system for the United States through which to review herbs. The presidential commission on dietary supplements recently recommended exactly this sort of system.

When Congress enacted DSHEA in 1994, this comprehensive piece of legislation established a new regulatory framework for supplements, ensuring continued access to safe products, made to quality standards. It also allowed for increased dissemination of information about the health benefits of these products. In signing the act, President Clinton declared, "we have finally reformed the way government treats consumers and supplements in a way that encourages good health."

Congress, in its findings, explained why it had chosen to pass this legislation:

- National surveys have revealed that almost 50% of the 260 million Americans regularly consume dietary supplements of vitamins, minerals, or herbs as a means of improving their nutrition

- Consumers should be empowered to make choices about preventive health-care programs based on data

from scientific studies of health benefits related to particular dietary supplements

- Legislative action that protects the right of access of consumers to safe dietary supplements is necessary in order
to promote wellness

- Dietary supplements are safe within a broad range of intake,
and safety problems with supplements are relatively rare

- Although the federal government should take swift action against products that are unsafe or adulterated, the
federal government should not impose unreasonable regulatory barriers limiting or slowing the flow of safe products and accurate information

- A rational federal framework must be established to su-
persede the current ad hoc, patchwork regulatory policy
on dietary supplements

## *Terms of DSHEA*

The legislation defined dietary supplements, created a
mechanism for dealing with safety issues, regulated health
claims and labeling of dietary supplements, provided for
good manufacturing practices, and established new government entities to review regulations and encourage research
on dietary supplements.

Dietary supplement ingredients may not be regulated
as food additives. A dietary supplement can be removed
from the market if the FDA shows that it presents "a significant or unreasonable risk of illness or injury." Truthful and
nonmisleading claims that describe the role of a nutrient
in supporting wellness will still be allowed on dietary supplement labels. (Examples: calcium builds strong bones;
antioxidants protect against cell damage.) These claims are
referred to as structure/function claims or nutritional support claims.

In some cases, the label may have to include the following disclaimer: "This statement has not been evaluated by the FDA. This product is not intended to diagnose, treat, cure, or prevent any disease." A product making this kind of claim may not be classified as a drug solely because of the claim.

This legislation maintains FDA authority to remove any unsafe product, but requires that the agency do it in a reasonable, methodical fashion. The legislation permits a new category of claims called "nutrition support" claims, which do not require FDA pre-authorization. These claims may describe the effect of a dietary supplement on the structure or function of the body, the biological mechanism by which a product acts, and effects on well-being.

Truthful informational materials, including articles in scientific journals, which present a balanced point of view and do not promote a specific company or brand of supplement, can be distributed by dietary supplement sellers as long as they are displayed separately from the supplements.

In the fall of 1997, in order to help consumers better understand and compare products, the FDA published final dietary supplement labeling regulations as required by DSHEA. The regulations, which will become effective in March 1999, state that: Dietary supplements are to be identified by the term "dietary supplement" as a part of the statement of identity; the "facts box" for dietary supplements will be titled "Supplement Facts" (for conventional foods, it is titled "Nutrition Facts"), and the part of the plant used in a product must be identified on the label for botanical ingredients.

# Perception Is Reality

In 1997, there were several incidents of misuse and abuse of the stimulant, antiasthma herb ephedra, and there was an

FDA move to declare it illegal. Some states actually banned its sale. The herbal industry defended the herb as traditionally used for 3,000 years. The FDA countered that such history was not as currently used, as a stimulant in huge dosages with a likelihood of abuse. When *Dateline NBC* interviewed the outspoken manufacturer of the ephedra product "Herbal Ecstasy," he seized his moment on camera to declare, "I've got something better than ephedra—kava!" All too often, perception becomes reality. From that moment on, in the minds of too many, kava was linked with ephedra and with abuse. An Association of Food & Drug Officials journal concluded that ". . . kava . . . may have an abuse potential similar to alcohol . . . [and that it was] being marketed as an alternative to alcohol."

The industry faces a critical challenge: To set high standards of quality, safety, marketing, and packaging in order to protect its future. In the words of esteemed ethnopharmacologist Varro Tyler, "If marketed responsibly, kava could become the anxiolytic of choice. Kava is such an effective herb, the FDA cannot afford to ignore it. If abuse occurs, or if claims are abusive, FDA will strike it down."[12] Rob McCaleb of Herb Research Foundation warns, "The FDA is uneasy about kava due to its being marketed as a mind-altering substance, and the FTC is looking hard at advertising claims."[13]

# Kava Council

If an opportunistic company comes along and markets a product with kava and makes wild claims that turn out to be false, it is possible for kava to be treated and regulated as a drug. Although kava is subtle and nonthreatening, most in the natural products industry fear its future could be fraught with danger if it is marketed as a psychoactive substance. A golden seal of approval from the FDA would go a long way toward enhancing public perception of the herb.

To this end, 30 manufacturers and suppliers have formed the Kava Committee, within and under the direct auspices of the American Herbal Products Association. The committee funded a "comprehensive study of the efficacy and safety of kava, peer-reviewed from a medical and legal perspective." Their goal is to make sure kava gets what the FDA terms a structure/function claim: the information and substantiation the FDA needs to allow the industry to make certain claims about kava products. It appears at this time that the kava industry is doing all the right things to assure its safe and successful emergence into the American mainstream.

## The Economic and Political Future of Kava

Kava has enormous potential as a new herb for the treatment of our present-day problems of stress, anxiety, and insomnia. The main stakeholders in this process are the pharmaceutical industry, the FDA, health practitioners and researchers, the public, the supplement industry (including exporters, importers, manufacturers, retail), and the growers. The availability of this valuable product, and its safe and effective use, depend on the cooperation of all these players, despite any differences in perception, needs, and goals.

## CHAPTER 18

# Closing
# Thoughts

Kava stands on its own as a unique herbal remedy for stress, anxiety, and insomnia. We have discussed when and how to use it, the research and clinical evidence of its actions and effectiveness, and how it compares favorably with prescription medications. There is also the broader perspective of its historic and cultural context, which suggests other possible uses. We find in this herb an unusual combination of safety and effectiveness, a broad range of positive effects, and lack of side effects. With the high cost of medical care and pharmaceuticals, and the increasing trend to self care, kava provides a low-risk/high-gain stress-relieving agent that is safe and easy to administer. Although my professional preference is that individuals avoid self-diagnosis and self-treatment, many may find that self-treatment with the herb is all they need.

Similar to its traditional use, kava also has a present-day role in conflict resolution. It promotes peaceful and "safe" communication, a very needed commodity on all levels—interpersonal, corporate, political, and even international. Kava also opens a window into a number of timely and complex issues, such as the origins and treatment of anxiety and stress, conventional vs. holistic approaches to (mental) health care, political and economic realities of kava production and regulation, and finally, kava's role in our relationship to nature.

## Solutions to Stress

Stress and anxiety are exacting enormous costs in many areas in our individual lives; our physical and mental health; our relationships, families, and organizations; and in society as a whole. Our consumption-oriented lifestyles create increasing stress and anxiety as we struggle to keep up with an ever-elusive goal. Is it more money, more things, more time, or more happiness that we seek? Do we even know what we want, let alone how to get it?

A common solution to stress-induced anxiety has often been to pop a pill. Our goal, however, is not to replace antianxiety medication with an herbal remedy. Rather, it is to examine the context of our disease and find a more deeply based solution, using kava as a bridge. Whether we call the natural approach to medical care holistic, alternative, integrative, orthomolecular, or complementary, it is the approach of the future. It is essential that, in medical care, we treat the whole person. No matter how natural and safe kava and other herbs may be, we still need to look for the root causes of disease, rather than just treating symptoms. For example, if a condition is psychologically based, it is important to explore issues and find psychological answers (see Chapter 4). If there is a metabolic or chemical imbalance anywhere in the body, it should be addressed as such (see Chapters 3 and 13). If the problems are related more to lifestyle, we have provided a few guiding principles and specific techniques for addressing them. Ideally, we can use our confrontation with the "stress problem" as a first step in exploring all aspects of the self, toward the goal of optimal health in mind, body, and spirit.

## The Future of Health Care

This is an exciting time to be a physician, with many new possibilities for healing. The success of herbs like kava are leading to a renewed recognition and acceptance of herbal and natural medicine. It is bringing this entire field to the attention of the general population, those who are willing to look beyond conventional medicine for solutions to health problems. Our dependence on technological medicine, including the use of pharmaceuticals, has not yielded increased freedom from disease.

I believe most doctors are motivated to find the best, least-harmful approaches to helping their patients. Many of my colleagues, previously skeptical of my interest and practice, now ask me for information on how to use a more natural approach. This field is growing so quickly it is difficult to keep up. Fortunately, patients who seek complementary care tend to be those most likely to take responsibility for their own healing, and least likely to expect the doctor to do everything or to know it all.

## The Politics of Addiction

Earlier, we addressed the issue of over-prescribing the antianxiety agents benzodiazepines (see Chapter 5). Here we will look at the larger issues of addiction, the pharmaceutical industry, and the industrialization of health care.

The nonaddictive aspect of kava spotlights the medical and societal problem of addiction to benzodiazepines. The profit motive is driving the popularity of these drugs, and danger lies not just in the addiction potential and other dangerous side effects, but in their use as a "societal hypnotic." The symptoms of our conditions are being tranquilized away. While some worry that kava is a potential substance of abuse, the truth is quite the opposite. In fact, in many ways it cam be seen as part of the solution, as we have seen throughout this book.

Using antianxiety agents to treat chronic anxiety is like using alcohol to treat "the shakes" from a bad hangover. It may work, but the hangover is not the real problem. The problem is the "one too many" you drank last night!

Researcher Kenneth Blum sees addiction as stemming from "reward deficiency," a genetic predisposition to insufficient stimulation in the brain by certain "feel good" transmitters (see Chapter 3). The individual may then use drugs or thrill-seeking behaviors, such as gambling, to artificially raise the neurotransmitter levels. This is only temporary, and when the brain is once again deprived of this stimulation, withdrawal sets in.

In his television special, *Close to Home,* Bill Moyers says the addictive substance "hijacks your brain." Your will and good sense are replaced by an overriding need for the addictive substance—whatever it may be—alcohol, tobacco, cocaine, or prescription drugs. These substances stimulate the pleasure receptors in the brain to relieve pain, including that caused by withdrawal, and even produce pleasure, but at a high cost. The user experiences temporary relief, but becomes a slave in the process. For example, when given a choice of drug or food buttons to push, rats will die of starvation in pursuit of a cocaine high.

Any way you look at it, addictiveness is the price of most "feel-good" chemicals, from the stimulants, such as nicotine, amphetamine, and cocaine to the more sedating compounds, such as heroin, barbiturates, and benzodiazepines. Soon (within a few weeks in the case of benzodiazepines), the user is taking the substances just to relieve the pain of not taking them! Though it appears in the fine print of their descriptive literature, the pharmaceutical industry, like the tobacco industry, does not prominently announce the addictiveness of their products.

The problem is undeniable, yet it continues daily. There is little objection from the victims—the addicted ones and their families—and certainly not from those they kill in car accidents while under the influence. Can we, as physicians, plead innocence? Just as the shaman or medicine man of the past was trusted to deliver the correct potion, today's physician is expected to prescribe the appropriate medicine. Too often, this does not happen, and everyone continues to look the other way, doctors included.

Are doctors too busy to actually listen to their patients and try to diagnose and treat their underlying problems? The answer, in most cases, is yes. And it pains many good physicians who no longer practice the *art* of medicine as healing.professionals. As a result of the industrialization of medical care, they have, of necessity, become pill-pushers. The HMOs, insurance companies, pharmaceutical companies, and hospital chains are big business, answerable to their stockholders to show a profit.

Despite such justified criticisms, it is difficult to blame anyone in particular. The truth is more likely in the words of the prophet Pogo, "We have met the enemy and it is us." We have allowed our lives to be co-opted by a profit-motivated economic structure of which the medical care system is but a part. In a system of competition and domination, we are alienated from each other and from nature. We are no longer the tribe that takes care of its own people and its environment the way the "primitives" have done. Kava is a step toward breaking this drug addiction and reconnecting with ourselves and with nature.

# Return to Nature

We can only truly ease our stress-related "diseases" if we acknowledge the social and cultural context in which the disease and the desired healing takes place. As Herbalist David Hoffmann so clearly declares, "It is a therapeutic and moral mistake to use herbal remedies to relieve our physical and physiological distress if we continue in patterns of thought, behavior, work, and culture that are themselves the source of the disease. We are at home on this planet—we have only to recognize it."[1]

We must connect back to the "real" system of which we are all part—the earth, the plants, the animals, and each other; first, by connecting back to ourselves; to our own hearts and souls. We need to step back from the "madding crowd," from our TVs, billboards, freeways, and urban jungles. We need to meditate and feel ourselves—in the quiet that is at our core. We need to override the pervasive programming of the marketplace, and begin to know who we really are and what we truly need and want.

Hoffmann continues with his suggested solution, "Through their power to alleviate the very ills of humanity, herbal remedies provide a clue, a signpost, to this reality: We are part of a wonderfully integrated whole. There is a wisdom in plants that can help us to regain ourselves and our health and wholeness. By attuning ourselves to the plants and their healing qualities, we establish a rapport with nature."[2] The herbalists and the medicine men and women have always understood the healing power of plants, this conduit back to ourselves and to the planet that nurtures us all—plant, animal, and human.

Individual plant species have their own specific gifts for us: Willow bark produces aspirin, foxglove yields digitalis, and periwinkle extract can treat leukemia. The list is nearly as extensive as our pharmacopeia, and will continue to grow. Parenthetically, it will become even longer if we preserve the rainforests long enough for thousands more species to be collected, analyzed, and utilized. This ancient plant knowledge is carried by the remaining tribal people, some of whom we had the privilege of meeting recently in the jungles of Ecuador. But we must hurry, as their culture and habitat are threatened daily with annihilation by oil, lumber, and cattle interests, for whom these remarkable people and their way of life are but an "inconvenience."

## Ethical Challenges Facing the Kava Industry

The issue of the keepers of the knowledge applies to kava as well. After all, our access to the gifts of kava come only through the diligence of the islanders who cultivated it over the centuries. Will the commercial use of kava simply make rich nations (or companies) richer, or will there be a payback to its native keepers (see Chapter 16)? With kava, we have an opportunity to help a Third World culture maintain itself with dignity and appropriate prosperity. The choices we make with regard to kava may tell us a great deal about ourselves, our world, and our future.

## Beyond the Solution to Stress: Pleasure and Quality of Life

Just as optimal health is more than the absence of disease, true mental health goes beyond the absence of anxiety or depression, to the enjoyment of pleasure for its own sake. This is not merely narcissistic self-absorption, nor the escape from reality that one finds in alcohol, but the starting point for a deeper connection with the self and spirit that arises from the traditional use of kava (see Chapter 6). While we may not be able to drink fresh kava from a shell on the islands, we can enjoy some of the benefits by taking the extract: conflict resolution, open communication, an enhanced meditative state, and a deeper connection with nature. Kava is not "for medicinal use only."

Kava can become a bridge between conventional and alternative therapies, and continue to open up the vast realm of natural treatments. This expanded approach can lead us full circle to an increased appreciation of our natural resources. Sustaining what we have and renewing what we have destroyed is our only hope for the future—of humanity, of all living beings on the planet.

We shall not cease from exploration
And the end to all our exploring
Will be to arrive where we started
And know the place for the first time.

—*T. S. Eliot,* Little Gidding

# APPENDIX A:
# RECOMMENDED READING

### Herbal Medicine, Supplements, and Nutrition

*Encyclopedia of Natural Medicine.* Michael Murray and Joseph Pizzorno. Rocklin, CA: Prima Publishing, 1994.

*Facts About Fats.* John Finnegan. Berkeley, CA: Celestial Arts, 1993.

*Fats That Heal, Fats That Kill.* Udo Erasmus. Blaine, WA: Alive Books, 1993.

*40-30-30 Diet.* Ann Louise Gittleman. New Canaan, CT: Keats Publishing, 1997.

*Healing Anxiety with Herbs.* Harold Bloomfield. New York, NY: HarperCollins, 1998.

*Mastering the Zone.* Barry Sears. New York, NY: Regan Books, 1997.

*Potatoes, Not Prozac.* Kathleen Desmaisons and Candace B. Pert. New York, NY: Simon & Schuster, 1998.

*The Real Vitamin and Mineral Book, 2nd Edition.* Shari Lieberman and Nancy Bruning. Garden City Park, NY: Avery Publishing Group, 1997.

*Stress & Natural Healing.* Christopher Hobbs. Loveland, CO: Interweave Press, 1997.

*Stress, Anxiety, and Insomnia.* Michael Murray. Rocklin, CA: Prima Publishing, 1995.

*Sugar Blues.* William Dufty. New York, NY: Warner Books, 1993.

*The Way Up From Down.* Priscilla Slagle. New York, NY: Random House, 1987.

### Alternative/Integrative Medicine

*Brain Longevity.* Dharma Singh Khalsa. New York, NY: Warner Books, 1997.

*8 Weeks to Optimum Health.* Andrew Weil. New York, NY: Alfred Knopf Publishing, 1997.

*Five Steps to Selecting the Best Alternative Medicine.* Mary and Michael Morton. New Novato, CA: World Library, 1996.

*Healing Through Nutrition.* Melvyn Werbach. New York, NY: Harper-Collins, 1994.

*Reclaiming Our Health.* John Robbins. Tiburon, CA: H.J. Kramer Publishing, 1997.

*Spontaneous Healing.* Andrew Weil. New York, NY: Alfred Knopf Publishing, 1995.

### Mind–Body Medicine and Psychotherapy

*Creativity.* Mikaly Czikszenthihalyi. New York, NY: HarperCollins, 1996.

*Embracing Your Inner Critic.* Hal and Sidra Stone. San Francisco, CA: HarperSan-Francisco, 1995.

*EMDR.* Francine Shapiro and Margot Silk Forrest. New York, NY: BasicBooks, 1997.

*Emotional Intelligence.* Daniel Goleman. New York, NY: Bantam Books, 1995.

*Healing and the Mind.* Bill Moyers. New York, NY: Doubleday, 1993.

*Molecules of Emotion.* Candace Pert. New York, NY: Scribner, 1997.

*Waking the Tiger Within.* Peter Levine. Berkeley, CA: North Atlantic Books, 1997.
*Why Zebras Don't Get Ulcers.* Robert Sapolsky. New York, NY: W.H. Freeman and Co., 1994.
*Minding the Body, Mending the Soul.* Joan Borysenko. New York, NY: Bantam Books, 1998.

## Lifestyle

*Everyday Blessings: The Inner Work of Mindful Parenting.* Jon and Myla Kabat-Zinn. New York, NY: Hyperion, 1997.
*The Pleasure Zone.* Stella Resnick. Berkeley, CA: Conari Press, 1997.
*Power Sleep.* James Maas. New York, NY: Villard, 1998.
*Real Power: Business Lessons from the Tao Te Ching.* James Autry and Stephen Mitchell. New York, NY: Riverhead Books, 1998.
*TIKHAL: The Continuation.* Ann and Alexander Shulgin. Berkeley, CA: Transform Press, 1997.
*Voluntary Simplicity.* Duane Elgin. New York, NY: William Morrow, 1993.
*Wherever You Go, There You Are.* Jon Kabat-Zinn. New York, NY: Hyperion Publishing, 1995.

## Women's Health

*Before the Change.* Ann Louise Gittleman. New York, NY: HarperCollins, 1997.
*Hormone Replacement Therapy, Yes or No.* Betty Kamen. Novato, CA: Nutrition Encounter, Inc., 1993.
*What Your Doctor May Not Tell You About Menopause.* John Lee. New York, NY: Warner Books, 1996.
*Women's Bodies, Women's Wisdom.* Christiane Northrup. New York, NY: Bantam, 1994.

## Other Kava Books

*Kava: Medicine Hunting in Paradise.* Chris Kilham. Rochester, VT: Park Street Press, 1996.
*Kava, Nature's Relaxant.* Hasnain Walji. Prescott, AZ: Holm Press, 1997.
*Kava: The Pacific Elixir.* Lebot, Vincent, Merlin, Mark, Lindstrom, Lamont. Rochester, VT: Healing Arts Press, 1992.

# APPENDIX B:
# RESOURCES

## Herbal Medicines

### INFORMATION

American Botanical Council
P.O. Box 201660
Austin, TX 78720
(512) 331-8868
Website: *www.herbalgram.org*

This organization provides education about the medicinal use of herbs. Their herbal education catalogue carries a comprehensive list of articles, books, tapes, and other resources. American Botanical Council publishes the translated German Commission E Report, and, together with the Herbal Research Foundation, publish the informative, well-illustrated quarterly, *Herbalgram.*

American Herbal Pharmacopeia
P.O. Box 5159
Santa Cruz, CA 95063
(408) 438-1700
(408) 461-6317 (fax)

This organization produces detailed, peer-reviewed monographs on the safe, effective use of various herbal medicines, and is distributed by the *Herbalgram.* The monographs on St. John's wort and kava were immensely helpful to me in writing my books on these subjects.

Herb Research Foundation
1007 Pearl Street, Suite 200
Boulder, CO 80302-9953
(303) 449-2265
(800) 748-2617
(303) 449-7849 (fax)
Website: *www.herbs.org*

This organization provides education and information on the medicinal use of herbs, including the National Healthcare Hotline on safe herb use.

Natural Product Research Consultants
(NPRC)
600 First Avenue, Suite 205
Seattle, WA 98104
(206) 623-2520
Website: *www.nprc.com*

Publishers of *Quarterly Review of Natural Medicine* and *Clinical Applications of Natural Medicine Monograph* series, for health care professionals; and *Herbal Prescriptions for Better Health,* for consumers.

Program for Collaborative Research in
the Pharmaceutical Sciences
M/C 877
College of Pharmacy—UIC
833 South Wood Street
Chicago, IL 60612
(312) 996-2246

## PRACTITIONERS

American Herbalists' Guild
P.O. Box 746555
Arvada, CO 80006
(303) 423-8800
(303) 423-8828 (fax)
Website: *www.healthy.com/herbalists*

Membership organization for herbalists provides names of practitioners.

## HERBAL SUPPLIERS— MAIL ORDER

Advanced Physicians Products
831 State Street
Santa Barbara, CA 93101
(800) 220-7687
(800) 438-6372 (fax)
E-mail: app@silcom.com
Website: *www.approducts.com*

Physician-formulated products; free mail-order catalog.

Elixir Tonics & Teas
8612 Melrose Avenue
Los Angeles, CA 90065
(888) 4-TONICS
(310) 657-9300
(310) 957-9311 (fax)
Website: *www.elixirnet.com*

Full elixir bar and herbal store; free mail-order catalog; consultations with licensed herbalist available in person and by phone.

## *Natural Medicine*

### INFORMATION

American College for Advancement in
  Medicine (ACAM)
P.O. Box 3427
Laguna Hills, CA 96253
(714) 583-7666
(800) 532-3688

This is an organization of doctors and osteopaths who practice orthomolecular medicine, chelation therapy, and preventive medicine.

### PRACTITIONERS

American Holistic Medical Association
  and American Holistic Nurses' Association
4101 Lake Boone Trail, Suite 201
Raleigh, NC 27607
(919) 787-5181
(800) 278-AHNA
(919) 787-4916 (fax)

American Medical Student Association
1902 Association Drive
Reston, VA 22091
(703) 620-6600
(703) 620-5873 (fax)

Canadian Holistic Medical Association
491 Eglinton Avenue West, #407
Toronto, Ontario Canada
M5N 1A8
(416) 485-3071

Center for Mind-Body Medicine
5225 Connecticut Avenue N.W., Suite
  414
Washington, DC 20015
(202) 966-7338
(202) 966-2589 (fax)

Holistic Health Directory
New Age Journal
42 Pleasant Street
Watertown, MA 02172
(617) 926-0200

Office of Alternative Medicine
9000 Rockville Pike
Building 31, Room 5B-37
Mailstop 2182
Bethesda, MD 20892
(301) 402-2466
(301) 402-4741 (fax)

## *Acupuncture and Chinese Medicine*

American Academy of Medical
  Acupuncture
5820 Wilshire Boulevard, Suite 500
Los Angeles, CA 90036
(213) 937-5514
(213) 937-0959 (fax)
E-mail: KCKD71F@ prodigy.com

American Association of Acupuncture
  and Oriental Medicine
433 Front Street
Catasauqua, PA 18032-2506
(610) 266-1433
(610) 264-2768 (fax)
Email: AAOM1@AOC.com

## *Biofeedback (Including Neurofeedback)*

AAPB
10200 West 44th Avenue, Suite 304
Wheat Ridge, CO 80033-2840
(303) 422-8436
(303) 422-8894 (fax)
E-mail: aapb@resourcenter.com
Website: *www.aapb.org/aapb.htm*

Contains books and related material.

# Appendix B: Resources    255

Flexyx, LLC
106 La Casa Via, Suite 110
Walnut Creek, CA 94598
(510) 906-0422
(510) 906-0419 (fax)
Website: *www.flexyx.com*

Neurotherapy systems and clinical consulting.

Futurehealth, Inc.
3171 Rail Avenue
Trevose, PA 19053
(215) 364-4445
(215) 364-4447 (fax)
Website: www.futurehealth.org

## Chiropractic Medicine

American Chiropractic Association
1701 Clarendon Boulevard
Arlington, VA 22209
(703) 276-8800
(800) 986-4636
(703) 243-2593 (fax)

International Chiropractors Association
1110 North Glebe Road, Suite 1000
Arlington, VA 22201
(703) 528-5000

Association for Network Chiropractic
444 Main Street
Longmont, CO 80501
(303) 678-8086

## Clinical Nutrition

International and American Associations of Clinical Nutritionists (IAACN)
5200 Keller Springs Road, Suite 410
Dallas, TX 75248
(972) 250-2829
(972) 250-0233 (fax)

## COMPOUNDING PHARMACIES

Most will ship anywhere in the country. They are also handy resources for referrals to alternative physicians.

International Academy of Compounding Pharmacists
(800) 927-4227

## ENVIRONMENTAL MEDICINE

American Academy of Environmental Medicine
10 East Randolph Street
New Hope, PA 18938
(215) 862-4544
(215) 862-4583 (fax)

Human Ecology Action League
P.O. Box 29629
Atlanta, GA 30359
(404) 248-1898

## Homeopathic Medicine

American Institute of Homeopathy
1503 Glencoe
Denver, CO 80220
(303) 898-5477

Homeopathic Educational Services
2124 Kittredge Street
Berkeley, CA 94704
(510) 649-0294
(510) 649-1955 (fax)
E-mail: mail@homeopathic.com
Website: *www.homeopathic.com*

## Naturopathic Medicine

American Association of Naturopathic Physicians
601 Valley Street, #105
Seattle, WA 98109
(206) 298-0125

Bastyr University of Natural Health Sciences
14500 Juanita Drive Northeast
Bothell, WA 98011
(425) 823-1300
(425) 823-6222 (fax)
E-mail: admiss@bastyr.edu
Website: *www.bastyr.edu*

The Canadian College of Naturopathic Medicine
2300 Yonge Street, 18th Floor, Box 2431
Toronto, Ontario Canada
M4P IE4
(416) 486-8584

National College of Naturopathic Medicine
11231 S.E. Market Street
Portland, OR 97216
(503) 255-4860
(503) 257-5929 (fax)

Southwest College of Naturopathic
Medicine and Health Sciences
6535 East Osborn Road, Suite 703
Scottsdale, AZ 85251
(602) 990-7424
(602) 990-0337 (fax)

Price-Pottenger Nutrition Foundation
P.O. Box 2614
La Mesa, CA 91943
(800) 366-3748

## Orthomolecular Psychiatry

Well Mind Association of Greater
Washington
11141 Georgia Avenue, #326
Wheaton, MD 20902
(301) 949-8282

This organization provides a regular
lecture series for the public, and referrals of alternative health practitioners.

## Osteopathic Medicine

American Academy of Osteopathy
3500 DePauw Boulevard, #1080
Indianapolis, IN 46268
(317) 879-1881

American Osteopathic Association
142 East Ontario Street
Chicago, IL 60611
(312) 280-5800

## Preventive Medicine

American Preventive Medical Association
459 Walker Road
Great Falls, VA 22066
(800) 230-2762

## Internet Resources

The following alternative-health sites
are in addition to those found in
other listings, and include my own
site. These are for informational purposes only. While we recommend
these sites, we are not endorsing any
sites in particular, or their products.

## HEALTH

*www.doctorcass.com* (Dr. Hyla Cass)

*www.healthy.net* (Health World Online)

Excellent resource for information,
practitioners, and speakers. Linked to
many other good sites, as well.

*www.drweil.com* (Ask Dr. Weil)

## KAVA

*www.coconut.com/features/kava.html*

Features on South Pacific culture, including kava, by Brian Dear

*www.vanuatu.net.vu/kava.htm*

A web page for Kava Kompani, a distributor and exporter of raw kava root
to herbal companies. Since they do
not sell to the general public, they re-
quest that consumers not e-mail kava
orders.

*www.silk.net/personal/scombs/kava.html*

Stan Combs's "Kava in Vanuatu"
page. A fascinating photo essay on the
history and ethnobotany of kava and
the ni-Vanuatu (as the people of Vanuatu are known). An excellent place to
start for those who are just beginning
the kava journey.

*www.kavapure.com*

Pure World Botanicals' Website has
color photos of Vanuatu peoples and
kava making.

*www.natrol.com*

Natrol's home page, containing white
papers on various herbs as well as information about their Kavatrol product.

*www.health-science.com/mela.htm*

An article on insomnia, melatonin,
and kava root extract.

*www.netstorage.com/kami/wwwboard/kav
abowl.html*

The Kava Bowl Web conferencing
forum.

*www.prairienet.org/~kagan/kavabib.html*

Lee Kagan's reference guide to everything you ever wanted to know about
kava. An invaluable tool for readers looking to find out more about the subject

# APPENDIX C:
# KAVA BEVERAGE
# PREPARATION RECIPE

Any herb supplier or health food store should have kava powder. If not, they should be able to order it for you. For those of you interested in preparing the kava beverage yourselves from powder, we describe two simple methods:

## Water Method

Wrap a cup of kava powder loosely in a piece of cloth.

Holding the edges of cloth loosely above the ball of kava, plunge the kava up and down in 4 cups of water, stopping occasionally to squeeze out the kava ball. Continue plunging it up and down until the water is a "coffee-and-cream" color. (This should take 5 to 15 minutes.) Drink!

## Emulsion Method

INGREDIENTS:

1 cup kava powder
4 cups water
6 tablespoons vegetable oil (I've used olive or canola)
2 tablespoons liquid lecithin.

Blend all ingredients at top speed for five minutes, until the liquid is "coffee-and-cream" colored. Strain liquid through a fiber filter. Since straining can take time (and patience), you may want to use something fairly loose, like cheesecloth. Eventually, all the liquid will drain out, leaving the solid ingredients in a ball in your strainer or cloth, and a bowl of suspicious smelling liquid. Once this happens, you can throw away the solid mass. Drink!

\* \* \*

There are a couple types of resins in the root, some of which are extracted using just water. There are others, which are not water soluble and need to be emulsified, hence the oil and lecithin extraction procedure. The emulsion method should release more kavalactones.

A couple of other notes about preparation: According to Vincent Lebot, when you grind kava to dry it, it loses some of its power. Freeze-drying the resinous, milk-like, non-water soluble emulsion preserves freshness. Lebot recommends against storing the liquid, since, like milk, it is an environment for bacterial growth. Dr. Asesela Ravuvu reminded us that in Kona, kava was traditionally ground and drunk fresh. According to him, dried kava came only with commercialization. In Fiji, dried kava is known as "dead" kava.

# NOTES

## CHAPTER 1

1. Nesse, R., M.D., and Williams, G., Ph.D., *Why We Get Sick*. New York, NY: Vintage Books, (1996): 212.
2. "Report of the National Commission on Sleep Disorders" *USA Today* (January 1993): 63.
3. Rosch, P., "Is Job Stress America's Leading Adult Health Problem? A Commentary" *Business Insights* (October 1991): 87.
4. Lehmann, E. et al., "Efficacy of a Special Kava Extract in Patients with States of Anxiety, Tension and Excitedness of Non-Mental Origin—A Double Blind Placebo Controlled Study of Four Weeks of Treatment" *Phytomedicine* (1996): 3: 113–119.
5. Astin, John A., "Why Patients Use Alternative Medicine" *Journal of the American Medical Association* (May 1998).
6. Harrisson, T. H., *Savage Civilization*, London: Gollancz, (1937): 275–280.

## CHAPTER 2

1. Ehrenreich, Barbara, *Blood Rites*. New York, NY: Metropolitan Publications,(1997): 78.
2. Cannon, Walter, "The Role of Emotion in Disease" *Annals of Internal Medicine* (May 1936): 9:2.
3. Seaward, Brian, *Managing Stress*. Sudbury, MA: Jones and Bartlett, (1997): 5.
4. Holmes, T., and Rahe, R., "The Social Readjustment Scale" *Journal of Psychosomatic Research* (1967): 11: 213–218.
5. Selye, Hans, M.D., *Stress Without Distress*. New York, NY: New American Library, (1974): 14.
6. Swenson, Richard, *Margin*. Colorado Springs, CO: Navpress, (1992): 60.
7. See note 5 above.
8. Tavris, Carol, "Coping With Anxiety" *Science Digest* (February 1986): 51.
9. DSM-IV, *Diagnostic and Statistical Manual of Mental Disorders, IV.* Washington, D.C.: American Psychiatric Association, (1994).
10. Drummond, Edward, M.D., *Overcoming Anxiety Without Tranquilizers*. New York, NY: Dutton Books, (1997): 40.
11. Hart, A., *Adrenaline and Stress*. Dallas, TX: Word Publishing, (1995): 48–49.

## CHAPTER 3

1. Nesse, R., M.D., and Williams, G., Ph.D., *Why We Get Sick*. New York, NY: Vintage Books, (1996): 213.

2. Nuernberger, Phil, Ph.D., *The Quest for Personal Power.* New York, NY: Putnam, (1996): 14–16.
3. Chopra, Deepak, *Quantum Healing: Exploring the Frontiers of Mind/Body Medicine.* New York, NY: Bantam Books, (1993): 134.
4. See note 2 above.

## CHAPTER 4

1. Crowe, R. et al., "A Family Study of Panic Disorder" *Archives of General Psychiatry* (1983): 40: 1065–1069.
2. Torgerson, S., "Genetic Factors in Anxiety Disorders" *Archives of General Psychiatry* (1983): 40: 1085–1089.
3. Levine, Peter, *Waking the Tiger Within.* Berkeley, CA: North Atlantic Books, (1997).
4. Shapiro, F., and Forrest, M., *EMDR.* New York, NY: Basic Books, (1997).
5. Stone, Hal and Stone, Sidra, *Embracing Your Inner Critic.* San Francisco, CA: HarperCollins, (1995).

## CHAPTER 5

1. Lader, M., "Dependence on Benzodiazepines" *Journal of Clinical Psychiatry* (1983): 44: 121–127.
2. Drummond, Edward, M.D., *Overcoming Anxiety Without Tranquilizers.* New York, NY: Dutton Books, (1997).
3. Oster, G. et al., "Benzodiazepine Tranquilizers and the Risk of Traffic Accidents" *American Journal of Public Health* (1990): 80: 1467–1470.
4. Tinetti, M.E. et al., "Risk Factors for Falls Among Elderly Persons Living in Community" *New England Journal of Medicine* (1988): 319: 1701–1707.
5. Cummings, S.R. et al., "Epidemiology of Osteoporosis and Osteoporotic Fractures" *Epidemiologic Review* (1985): 7: 178–208.
6. Lader, M. "Benzodiazepines: The Opiate of the Masses?" *Neuroscience* (1978): 3: 159–165.
7. Breggin, Peter, *Talking Back to Prozac.* New York, NY: St. Martin's Paperback ,(1995).
8. Gordon, Barbara, *I'm Dancing As Fast As I Can.* New York, NY: Harper & Rowe, (1976).
9. See note 6 above.

## CHAPTER 6

1. Theroux, Paul, *The Happy Isles of Oceania.* New York, NY: Putnam, (1992): 42.
2. Forster, J.G., *A Voyage Round the World in His Britannic Majesty's Sloop, Resolution.* London: J. White, (1777): 2: 150–189.
3. Ellis, W., *Polynesian Researches.* London: F. Gisher, Son and Jackson, (1828): 1: 229–231.
4. Hocart, A.M., *Lau Islands, Fiji.* Honolulu: Bishop Museum Bulletin, No. 75, (1929): 59–70.
5. Lemert, E.M., "Secular Use of Kava in Tonga" *Quarterly Journal of Studies on Alcohol* (1967): 18: 328–341.
6. British Herbal Medicine Association, *British Herbal Pharmacopeia* (1983).
7. Holmes, L., "The Function of Kava in Modern Samoan Culture" Ethnopharmacologic Search for Psychoactive Drugs, ed. Efron, D.H., et al, Washington, DC: Public Health Service Publications, (1967): 1645: 109.
8. See note 1 above.
9. Lebot, Vincent, Merlin, Mark, and Lindstrom, Lamont, *Kava: The Pacific Elixir.* Rochester, VT: Healing Arts Press, (1997).

## CHAPTER 7

1. Lebot, Vincent, Merlin, Mark, and Lindstrom, Lamont, *Kava: The Pacific Elixir.* Rochester, VT: Healing Arts Press, (1997).

2. Van Veen, A.G., "Isolation and Constitution of the Narcotic Substance from Kawa Kawa" *Receuil des Travaux Chimiques de Pays-Bas* (1939): 58: 521–527.
3. Steinmetz, E.F., *Kava Kava: Famous Drug Plant of the South Sea Islands.* San Francisco, CA: Level Press, (1960, 1961).
4. See note 1 above.
5. Klohs, M.W., et al., "A Chemical and Pharmacological Investigation of Piper Methysticum Forst" *J Me Pharm Chem* (1959) 1: 95–103.
6. Cheng, D., Lidgard, R.O., Duffield, P.H., Duffield, A.M., and Brophy, J.J., Biomedical Mass Spectrometry Unit, University of New South Wales, Kensington, Australia.
7. Shulgin, A., *The Narcotic Pepper—The Chemistry and Pharmacology of* Piper Methsticum *and Related Species.* Bulletin on Narcotics, (April–June 1973): 25: 59–74.
8. See note 1 above.
9. Duve R.N., *Gas-Liquid Chromatographic Determination Of Major Constituents of Piper Methysticum Analyst.* (1981): 106: 160–165.
10. Smith, et al., "High-Performance Liquid Chromatography of Kava Lactones" *Journal of Chromatography* (1984): 283: 303–308.
11. See note 3 above.
12. Pert, Candace, *Molecules of Emotion.* New York, NY: Scribner, (1997).
13. Jamieson, D.D. and Duffield, P.H., "The Antinociceptive Action of Kava Components in Mice" *Clinical and Experimental Pharmacology and Physiology* (1990): 17: 495–508.
14. Holm, E., et al., "Studies on the Profile of the Neurophysiological Effects of D,L-kavain: Cerebral Sites of Action and Sleep-Wakefulness-Rhythm in Animals" *Arzneim Forsch* (1991): 41: 673–83.
15. Davies, L., Drew, C., Duffield, P., and Jamieson, D., "Kavapyrones and Resin: Studies on GABA, GABA b and Benzodiazepine Receptor Sites in Rodent Brain" *Pharmacology and Toxicology* (1992): 71(2): 120–126.
16. Jussofie, A., Schmiz, A., Hiemke, C., "Kavapyrone Enriched Extract from Piper Methysticum as Modulator of the GABA Binding Site in Different Regions of Rat Brain" *Psychopharmacology* (1994): 469–474.
17. Meyer, H.J., and Kretzchmar, R., *Klin Wschr* (1966): 44, 902.
18. Meyer, H.J., "Pharmakologie der Wirksamen Prinzipien DES Kawa-Rhizoms" *Archives Internationales de Pharmacodynamie* (1962): 138: 505–536.
19. Singh, Y.N., "Effects of Kava on Neuromuscular Transmission and Muscle Contractility" *Journal of Ethnopharmacology* (1983): 7: 267–276.
20. Seitz, U., Ameri, A., Pelzer, H., et al., "Relaxation of Evoked Contractile Activity of Isolated Guinea-Pig Ileum by (+/-)-Kavain" *Planta Med* (1997): 63: 303–306.
21. See note 13 above.
22. Gleitz, J., Beile, A., and Peters, T., "(+/-)-Kavain Inhibits Veratridine-Activated Voltage-Dependent Na(+)- Channels in Synaptosomes Prepared from Rat Cerebral Cortex" *Neuropharmacology* (September 1995): 34(9): 1133–1138.
23. Magura E.I., et al., "Kava Extract Ingredients, (+)-Methysticin and (+/-)-Kavain Inhibit Voltage-Operated Na(+)-Channels in Rat CA1 Hippocampal Neurons" *Neuroscience* (1997): 81(2): 345–351.
24. Backhaus, C., Krigelstein, J., "Neuroprotective Activity of Kava Extract (Piper Methysticum) and Its Methysticin Constituents In Vivo and In Vitro" *Pharmacology of Cerebral Ischemia; Eur J Pharmac* (1992): 215: 265-269.
25. See note 4 above.
26. Keledjian J., Duffield, P.H., Jamieson, D.D., et al., "Uptake into Mouse Brain of Four Compounds Present in the Psychoactive Beverage Kava" *J Pharm Sci* (1988): 77: 1003–1006.

## CHAPTER 8

1. Volz, H.P. et al., "Kava-Kava Extract WS 1490 versus Placebo in Anxiety Disorders—A Randomized Placebo-Controlled 25 Week Outpatient Trial" *Pharmacopsychiatry* (1997): 30 (1): 1–5.

2. Lehmann, E., Kinzler, E., and Friedemann, J., "Efficacy of a Special Kava Extract in Patients with States of Anxiety, Tension and Excitedness of Non-Mental Origin—A Double Blind Placebo Controlled Study of Four Weeks of Treatment." *Phytomedicine Vol. III* (1996): 113–119.

3. Warnecke, G., "Psychosomatic Dysfunctions in the Female Climacteric: Clinical Effectiveness and Tolerance of Kava Extract WS 1490" *Fortschr Med* (1991): 109 (4): 119–122.

4. Warnecke G. et al., "Wirksamkeit von Kawa-Kawa-Extract beim klimakterischen Syndrom." *Z Phytother* (1990): 11: 81–86.

5. Lehmann, E., Klieser, R., Klimke, H. et al., "The Effects of Kavain on Patients Suffering from Anxiety" *Pharmacopsychiatry* (1989): 22: 258–262.

6. Münte, T.F., Heinze, H.J., Matzke, M., and Steitz, J., "Effects of Oxazepam and an Extract of Kava Root (Piper methysticum) on Event-Related Potentials in a Word-Recognition Task" *Neuropsychobiology* (1993): 27 (1): 46–53.

7. Woelk H., et al., "Double-Blind Study: Kava Extract versus Benzodiazepines in Treatment of Patients Suffering from Anxiety" *Z Allg Med* (1993): 69: 271–277.

8. Lindenberg, D. et al., "Kavain in Comparison with Oxazepam in Anxiety Disorders: A Double-Blind Study of Clinical Effectiveness" *Fortschr Med* (1990): 108: 49–50.

9. Singh, Y.N., "Effects of Kava on Neuromuscular Transmission and Muscle Contractility" *Journal of Ethnopharmacology* (1983): 7: 267–276.

10. Bruggenmann, F., et al., "Die analgetische Wirkung der Kawa-Inhaltsstoffe Dihydrokawain und Dihydromethysticin" *Arnzneim-Forsch* (1963): 13: 407–409.

11. Morrison, J., *The Journal of James Morrison.* London: Golden Cockerel Press, (1935): 151.

12. Carper, J., *Miracle Cures.* New York, NY: HarperCollins (1997): 160–161.

13. See note 3 above.

14. See note 4 above.

15. Baldi, D., "Sulle Propierta Farmacologische Del I Piper Methysticum" *Terapia Moderna* (1980): 4: 359-364.

16. Lebot, Vincent, Merlin, Mark, and Lindstrom, Lamont, *Kava: The Pacific Elixir.* Rochester, VT: Healing Arts Press, (1997).

17. Hansel, R. et al., "Characterization and Physiological Activities of Some Kava Constituents" *Pacific Science* (1966): 22: 293.

18. Hansel, R. et al., "Fungistatic Effects of Kava" *Planta Med* (1966): 14: 1–9.

19. Duffield, A.M. et al, *Journal of Chromatography* (1989): 475, 273.

20. Rasmussen, A.K. et al., "Metabolism of Some Kava Pyrones in the Rat" *Xenobiotica* (1979): 9: 1–16.

## CHAPTER 9

1. Gallup Organization, *Sleep in America: A National Survey of U.S. Adults,* poll conducted for the National Sleep Foundation. Princeton, N.J.: National Sleep Foundation, (1998).

2. Coren, Stanley, *Sleep Thieves.* New York, NY: Free Press, (1996).

3. NSF, *Drowsy Driving Fact Sheet.* Washington, DC: NSF, (1995).

4. Gallup Organization, *Sleep in America: A National Survey of U.S. Adults,* poll conducted for the National Sleep Foundation. Princeton, N.J.: National Sleep Foundation, (1995).

5. National Commission on Sleep Disorders Research, *Report of the National Commission on Sleep Disorders Research,* submitted to the U.S. Congress and to the secretary of the U.S. Department of Health and Human Services. (1993).

6. See note 4 above.

7. See note 1 above.

8. See note 1 above.

9. Krueger, J. M., and Mne hunting ajde, J. A., "Sleep as a Host Defense: Its Regulation by Microbial Products and Cytokines" *Clinical Immunology and Immunopathology* (1990): 188–199.

10. Irwin, M. et al., *Journal of The Federation of American Societies for Experimental Biology* (1996): 10: 643–653.
11. Pack, Allan, Medical Director, Washington, D.C.: National Sleep Foundation, (1996).
12. Segell, M., "The Secrets of Sleep" *Esquire* (October 1994).
13. See note 1 above.
14. See note 5 above.
15. See note 5 above.
16. See note 5 above.
17. Sandyk, R., "Melatonin and Maturation of REM Sleep" *International Journal of Neuroscience* (1992): 63: 105–114.
18. Reiter, F., and Robinson, J., *Your Body's Natural Wonder Drug, Melatonin.* New York, NY: Bantam Books (1995).
19. Gillin, J.C., "The Long and the Short of Sleeping Pills" *New England Journal of Medicine* (1991): 324 (24): 1725–1737.
20. Oster, G., Huse, D.M., Adams, S.F., Imbimbo, J., and Russell, M.W., "Benzodiazepine Tranquilizers and the Risk of Accidental Injury" *American Journal of Public Health* (1990): 80: 1467–1470.
21. Neutel, C.I., "Risk of Traffic Accident Injury After a Prescription for a Benzodiazepine" *Annals of Epidemiology* (1995): 5: 239–244.
22. Cook, P.J., Huggett, A., Graham-Pole, R., Savage, I.T., and James, I.M., "Hypnotic Accumulation and Hangover in Elderly Inpatients: A Controlled Double-Blind Study of Temazepam and Nitrazepam" *British Medical Journal* (1983): 286: 100–102.
23. Ray, W.A., Fought, R.L., and Decker, M.D., "Psychoactive drugs and the Risk of Injurious Motor Vehicle Crashes in Elderly Drivers" *American Journal of Epidemiology* (1992): 136 (70): 873–883.
24. Cummings, S.R., Kelsey, J.L., Nevitt, M.C., O'Dowd, K.J., "Epidemiology of Osteoporosis and Osteoporotic Fractures" *Epidemiologic Review* (1985): 7: 178–208.
25. Melton, L.J., Riggs, B.L., "Epidemiology of Age-Related Fractures" *The Osteoporotic Syndrome: Detection, Prevention, and Treatment* Stratton, New York: Grune and Stratton, (1983) : 45–72.
26. Tinetti, M.E., Speechley, M., and Ginter, S.F., "Risk Factors for Falls Among Elderly Persons Living in the Community" *New England Journal of Medicine* (1988): 319: 1701–1707.
27. Macdonald, J.B., "The Role of Drugs in Falls in the Elderly" *Clinics in Geriatric Medicine* (1985): 1 (3): 621–636.
28. Ray, W.A., Griffin, M.R., Schaffner, W., Baugh, D.K., and Melton, J., "Psychotropic Drug Use and the Risk of Hip Fracture" *New England Journal of Medicine* (1987): 316: 363–369.
29. Gales, B.J., and Mernard, S.M., "Relationship Between the Administration of Selected Medications and Falls in Hospitalized Elderly Patients" *Annals of Pharmacotherapy* (1995): 29: 354–358.
30. Gillin, J.C., "The Long and the Short of Sleeping Pills" *New England Journal of Medicine* (1991): 324 (24): 1725–1737.
31. Schneidrer-Helmert, D., "Why Low-Dose Benzodiazepine-Dependent Insomniacs Can't Escape Their Sleeping Pills" *Acta Psychiatricia Scandinavia* (1988): 78: 706–711.
32. Maquet, F.A., Dive, D., Salmon, E. et al., "Cerebral Glucose Utilization During Sleep-Wake Cycle in Man Determined by Positron Emission Tomography and [18F]2-Flouro-2-Deoxy-D-Glucose Method" *Brain Research 513* (1990): 136–143.
33. Smith, Carlyle and Lapp, Lorelei, "Increases in Number of REMs and REM Destiny in Humans Following an Intensive Learning Period" *Sleep* (1991): (14): 325–330.
34. Dujardin, Kathy, Guerrien, Alan, and Leconte, Pierre, "Sleep, Brain Activation, and Cognition" *Physiology and Behavior 47* (1990): 1271–1278.
35. Peterson, C., *Psychology: A Biopsychosocial Approach.* New York, NY: Longman (1997).
36. Hobson, J. Allan, *Sleep.* New York, NY: Scientific American Library, (1989).

37. Hammon, A. Christopher, *Getting More REM Sleep Contributes to Waking Up in a Good Mood.* Center for Sleep and Stress.
38. Lebot, Vincent, Merlin, Mark, and Lindstrom, Lamont, *Kava: The Pacific Elixir.* Rochester, VT: Healing Arts Press, (1997): 59.
39. Lebot, Vincent, *Les kavas en Oceanie: Etude Pluridisciplinaire D'une Culture Traditionnelle*, 1988.
40. Emser, W. and Bartylla, K., "Effect of Kava Extract WS 1490 on the Sleep Pattern in Healthy Subjects" *Neurologie/Psychiatrie* (1991): 5: 636-42.
41. Los Angeles Times, *Biological Psychiatry* (May 1998): 4.
42. Pierpaoli, Walter, Regelson, William, Colman, Carol, *The Melatonin Miracle.* New York, NY: Pocket Books, (1996).
43. McClusky, H.V., Milby, J.B., Switzer, P.K., Williams, V., and Wooten, V., "Efficacy of Behavioral Versus Triazolam Treatment in Persistent Sleep-Onset Insomnia" *American Journal of Psychiatry* (1991): 148: 121–126.
44. Milby, J.B., Williams, V., Hall, J.N., Khuder, S., McGill, T., and Wooten, V., "Effectiveness of Combined Triazolam-Behavioral Therapy for Primary Insomnia" *American Journal of Psychiatry* (1993): 150: 1259–1260.

## CHAPTER 10

1. Levine, Peter, as quoted by Brian Dear in his web report, "The Taste of Money" *www.coconut.com/features/kava.html.*
2. Blumenthal, Mark, Greunwald, Joerg et al., *The German Commission E. Monographs.* Austin, TX: American Botanical Council, (1998).

## CHAPTER 11

1. Almeida, J.C., Grimsley, E.W., "Coma from the Health Food Store: Interaction Between Kava Andalprazolam" *Ann Intern Med* (1996): 125: 940–941.
2. Jamieson, D.D. et al., "Positive Interaction of Ethanol and Kava Resin in Mice" *Clin and Exp Pharm and Phys* (1990): 17: 509–514.
3. Smith et al., "High-Performance Liquid Chromatography of Kava Lactones" *Journal of Chromatography* (1984): 283: 303–308.
4. Herberg, K.W., "Effect of Kava-Special Extract WS 1490 Combined with Ethyl Alcohol on Safety Relevant Performance Parameters" *Blutalkaohol* (1993): 30: 96–105.
5. Meyer, H.J., eds. Efron, D.H., Holmstead, B., Kline, N.S., *Pharmacology of Kava in Ethnopharmacologic Search for Psychoactive Drugs.* New York, NY: Raven Press, (1979): 133.
6. Hansel, Keller, Schneider, *Pharmaceutical Handbook.* Verlag: Springer, (1994): 210–221.
7. See note 6 above
8. Hoffmann, R. and Winter, U., "Therapeutic Observation with a Standardized Kava Extract" *V. Phytotherapiekongress; Bonn.* (November 1993).
9. Schulz, V., Hansel, R., Tyler, V., *Rational Phytotherapy.* New York, NY: Springer (1997): 71.
10. Gruenwald, J., Presentation at International Conference, 1996.
11. Russell, P., Bakker, D., Singh, N., "The Effects of Kava on Alerting and Speed of Access of Information form of Long Term Memory. *Bulletin of the Psychonomic Society* (1987): 25.
12. Volz, H.P. et al., "Kava-Kava Extract WS 1490 Versus Placebo in Anxiety Disorders—a Randomized Placebo-Controlled 25-Week Outpatient Trial" *Pharmacopsychiatry* (1997): 30 (1): 1–5.
13. Volz, H.P., Interview in *Clinical Pearls News* (July 1997).
14. Kinzler E., Kromer, J., Lehmann, E., "Effect of a Special Kava Extract in Patients with Anxiety, Tension, and Excitation States of Non-Psychotic Genesis. Double Blind Study with Placebos Over 4 Weeks" *Arzneimittelforschung* (1991): 41 (6): 584–588.
15. Lehmann, E. et al., "Efficacy of a Special Kava Extract in Patients with States of Anxiety, Tension, and Excitedness of Non-Mental Origin—A Double Blind

Placebo Controlled Study of Four Weeks of Treatment" *Phytomedicine* (1996): 113–119.

16. Norton, S.A., Ruze, P., "Kava Dermopathy" *J Am Acad Dermatol* (1994): 31: 89–97.
17. Shulgin, A., "The Narcotic Pepper—The Chemistry and Pharmacology of Piper Methsticum and Related Species" *Bulletin on Narcotics* (April–June 1973) 25: (2): 59–74.
18. Lebot, Vincent, Merlin, Mark, and Lindstrom, Lamont, *Kava: The Pacific Elixir.* Rochester, VT: Healing Arts Press, (1997).
19. Pfeiffer, et al., "Effects of Kava in Normal Subjects and Patients" *Efron Op.Cit.* (1967): 155–161.
20. Garner, L.F., Klinger, J.D., "Some Visual Effects Caused by the Beverage Kava" *Journal of Ethnopharmacology* (July 1985): 13(3): 307–311.
21. See note 13 above.
22. See note 14 above.
23. Warnecke G., "Psychosomatic Dysfunctions in the Female Climacteric: Clinical Effectiveness and Tolerance of Kava Extract WS 1490" *Fortschr Med* (1991): 109 (4): 119–122.
24. Duffield, P.H., Jamieson, D., School of Physiology and Pharmacology, University of NSW, Kensington, Australia, "Development of Tolerance to Kava in Mice" *Clinical and Experimental Pharmacology and Physiology* (1991): 18: 571–578.
25. William Gunn, *The Gospel of Futuna.* London: Hodder & Stoughton, (1914).
26. Mathews, J.D., Riley, M.D., Fejo, L. et al., "Effects of a Heavy Usage of Kava on Physical Health: Summary of a Pilot Survey in an Aboriginal Community." *Med J Aust* (1988): 148: 548–555.
27. Singh and Blumenthal, "Kava Monograph" *American Botanical Council* (1997) 39: 33–37.
28. Schelosky, L., Raffauf, C., Jendroska, K., Poewe, W., of the neurology department at Rudolf Virehote University in Berlin, "Letter to the Editor" *J. Neurol Neurosurg Psychiatry* (1995): 45: 639–640.

## CHAPTER 12

1. Linde, K. et al., "St. John's Wort for Depression: An Overview and Meta-Analysis of Randomized Clinical Trials" *BMJ* (1996): 313: 253–258.
2. Leathwood, P.D., "Aqueous Extract of Valerian Reduces Sleep Latency" *Planta Medica* (1985): 54: 144–148.
3. Leathwood, P.D., "Aqueous Extract of Valerian Improves Sleep Quality" *Pharmaco Biochem Behav* (1982): 17: 65–71.
4. Dressing, H., "Insomnia: Are Valerian/Balm Combinations of Equal Value to Benzodiazepine?" *Therapiewoch* (1992): 42: 726–736.
5. Hobbs, Christopher, *Stress and Natural Healing.* Santa Cruz, CA: Botanica Press, (1997).
6. Nirbhay, S., Professor of Psychiatry and Pediatrics at the Medical College Of Virginia, and Director of Commonwealth Institute for Child and Family Studies, Virginia Commonwealth University.
7. Nirbhay, S., Ph.D., and Ellis, C., M.D., "Kavatrol™ Reduces Daily Stress and Anxiety in Adults" Virginia Commonwealth University, unpublished study (1998).
8. Singh, Y., "Kava: An Overview" *Journal of Ethnopharmacology* (1992) 1: 13-45.
9. Singh, Y., "Effects of Kava on Neuromuscular Transmission and Muscle Contractility" *Journal of Ethnopharmacology* (1983): 267–276.

## CHAPTER 13

1. Hodges, R. et al., "Clinical Manifestation of Ascorbic Acid Deficiency in Man" *Am J C Nutr* (1971): 24: 432–43.
2. Cheraskin, E., *Vitamin C—Who Needs It?* Birmingham, AL: Arlington Press, (1993).
3. Clark, L.C., "Effects of Selenium Supplementation for Cancer Prevention" *JAMA* (1996): 276 (24): 1957–1963.

4. Gallup Organization, *Sleep in America: A National Survey of U.S. Adults,* poll conducted for the National Sleep Foundation. Princeton, N.J.: National Sleep Foundation, (1998).

## CHAPTER 14

1. Peterson, Karen S., "Working Hours are Longer, But Workplaces Seem Nicer" *USA Today* (April 1998).
2. Furchtgott-Roth, Diana (American Enterprise Institute), "Comp Time: Giving Hourly Workers What Money Can't Buy" National Center for Policy Analysis (April 1998).
3. Kabat-Zinn, Jon, *Wherever You Go, There You Are.* New York, NY: Hyperion, 1995.

## CHAPTER 15

1. Toren, C., "Making the Present, Revealing the Past: The Mutability and Continuity of Tradition as Process" *Man* (1988).
2. Harrisson, T. H., *Savage Civilization,* London: Gollancz (1937): 275–280.
3. Carleton Gajdusek, *Recent Observations on the Use of Kava in the New Hebrides, Ethnopharmacological Search for Psychoactive Drugs Symposium.* San Francisco, CA: U.S. Government, (1967).
4. Lemert, E.M., "Secular Use of Kava in Tonga" *Quarterly Journal of Studies on Alcohol* (1967): 328–341.
5. Kline, Nathan, *Recent Observations on the Use of Kava in the New Hebrides, Ethnopharmacological Search for Psychoactive Drugs Symposium.* San Francisco, CA: U.S. Government, (1967).
6. Herberg, K.W., "Fahrtuchtigkeit nach Einnahme von Kava-Spezial-Extract WS 1490" *Zeitschr. Allemein. Med.* (1991): 67: 842.
7. Weil, Andrew, *The Natural Mind.* Boston, MA: Houghton Mifflin, (1972): 23.

## CHAPTER 16

1. Ravuvu, Asesela, Live Presentation, The First International Botanical Symposium on Kava (1997).
2. Lebot, Vincent, Merlin, Mark, and Lindstrom, Lamont, *Kava: The Pacific Elixir.* Rochester, VT: Healing Arts Press, (1997).
3. Lebot, Vincent, Live Presentation, The First International Botanical Symposium on Kava (1997).
4. Kilham, Chris, *Kava Medicine Hunting in Paradise.* Rochester, VT: Inner Traditions, (1996): 54.
5. See note 3 above.
6. Khor, Martin, "Biotechnology: 'Gold Rush' Long Over, But 'Gene Rush' Is On" *Christian Science Monitor* (May 1997).
7. Lippert, Owen (Canada's Fraser Institute), "Pirates Plunder Patents. Will the Rule of Law Prevail?" *Wall Street Journal* (April 1998).

## CHAPTER 17

1. The Herbal Medical Data Base, *Who's Who in the World Herbal Medical Industry.* London: Alpine, Thorpe, and Warrier Limited, (1993).
2. Institute of Medical Statistics,. "Botanicals: A Role in US Health Care?" *Eaves M: The European Experience.* Washington (1994).
3. Haas, H., "Arzneipflanzenkunde. BI-Wiss-Verlag" *Mannheim* (1991): 1–196.
4. Farnsworth, N.R., Morris, R.W., "Higher Plants the Sleeping Giant of Drug Development" *American Journal of Pharmacy* (1976): 148: 46–52.
5. Leaders, Floyd, Live Presentation, The First International Botanical Symposium on Kava (1997).
6. "Survey on Use of Herbs in America", *Prevention* (1997).
7. Blumenthal, Mark, "Herb Sales Up 35% in Mass Market" *The Journal of the American Botanical Council and the Herb Research Foundation* (1995): 34.

8. Lancet Editorial Review, "Pharmaceuticals from Plants: Great Potential, Few Funds" *The Journal of the American Botanical Council* and the Herb Research Foundation (1995).

9. The Hartman & New Hope study is part of a larger four-part survey called "U.S. Consumer Use of Vitamins, Minerals and Herbal Supplements" in progress.

10. Meyer, H., "The Pills That Ate Your Profits," *Hospitals & Health Networks* (February 1998).

11. See note 5 above.

12. Tyler, Varro, Live Presentation, The First International Botanical Symposium on Kava (1997).

13. Mccaleb, Rob, Live Presentation, The First International Botanical Symposium on Kava (1997).

## CHAPTER 18

1. Blum, K., and Trachtenberg, M.C., "Addicts May Lack Some Neurotransmitters" *The U.S. Journal* (July 1987).

2. Hoffmann, David, *An Herbal Guide to Stress Relief.* Boulder Creek, CA: Planetary Arts Press, (1986).

# INDEX

**A**

Aalbersberg, Dr. William, 208, 226
Aborigines, Australian, 152
Accidents, automobile, 112
Adaptogens, 162–166
Addiction
  kava, 151–152
  politics, 245–248
  stress, 5
Adrenal glands
  function, 20, 22
  stress, 180–186
Adrenaline, 20
Agriculture
  bioengineering, 223–225
  economics, 217–220, 225–226
  Fiji, 220–222
  Hawaii, 222–223
  obstacles, 218–220
  opportunities, 218–220
  protecting, 226–228
  Vanuatu, 220–222
Alarm reaction, 21
Alcohol
  health and, 188–189
  kava interactions, 145
  kava *vs.*, 77
Alcoholics Anonymous, 188–189, 200
Alternative medicine, 8
American Heart Association, 33
American Psychiatric Association, 121
Americans
  alternative medicine, 8
  diet, 171–172
  herbal medicine
    consumption, 237–238

    interest, 231–233
  lifestyles, 191–194
    sleep and, 130–131
    stress study, 193–194
    work ethic, 113–114
Amino acids, 178–179
Analgesic effect, 88–90, 101–102
Anesthesia, local, 107–108
*Annals of Internal Medicine,* 181
Antioxidants, 173
Antidepressants
  description, 54–58
  side effects, 62–63, 157
Anxiety
  brain chemistry, 29–35
  case studies, 44–48, 59–61
  description, 23
  disorders
    incidence, 23–24
    types, 23–25
  genetic factors, 41–42
  medical causes, 38–39
  PTSD-induced, 43–44
  symptoms, 26
  treatments
    antidepressants, 54–58
    benzodiazepines, 58–59
    kava, 86–87
      clinical studies, 96–101
    natural, 65–66
Ascorbic acid, *see* Vitamin C
*As Good As It Gets,* 25
Ashwaganda, 164
Aspartame, 187
Attitude, 201–203
Awareness, 194–195

**B**
*Before the Change,* 105
Behavior, *see* Lifestyles
Being in present, 198–200
Benzodiazepines, *see also specific drugs*
    addiction, 123–125
    descriptions, 58–59
    elderly use, 122–124
    kava interaction, 143
    kava *vs.,* 99–100
    side effects, 62–63, 121–122
    tolerance, 123–125
    use, 121–125
"Benzodiazepines: The Opium of the
    Masses," 64
Bioengineering, 223–225
Biofeedback, 201
*The BioTech Century,* 223
Bladder infections, 110
Blum, Ken, 246
Blumenthal, Mark, 94–95, 232
Boron, 177
Botany, 69–70
Brain
    glucose metabolism, 125
    response system, 20, 22
    waves, 116
*Brave New World,* 211
Breathing, 200–201
Breggin, Peter, 62
*British Medical Journal,* 158
Brown, Dr. Donald, 159, 231
Burns, David, 23
Busse, Dr. Werner, 144

**C**
Caffeine, 189
Calcium, 177
Canadian Association of Herbal Prac-
    titioners, 69
Cannon, Walter, 14, 21
Carbohydrates, 179–180
Cayenne, 166
CFS, *see* Chronic fatigue syndrome
Children, 105–106
Chlorinated water, 187
Chopra, Deepak, 36–37
Christian, William, 145
Christian missionaries, 78–79
Chronic anxiety, 25–26
Chronic fatigue syndrome, 107
Cigarettes, *see* Smoking
Clinton, Hillary, 76
*Close to Home,* 246
Cobalamin, 174
Cocaine, 107–108

Commission E
    FDA *vs.,* 231
    monograph
        availability, 236–237
        description, 94–95
        kava report, 96–97
        kava safety, 141–142
        kava side effects, 147–148
Conflict resolution, 207–209
Consciousness, 213–214
Contraindications, 142
Convention on Biological Diversity,
    227–228
Convulsants, 101–102
Convulsions, 88–90
Cook, Captain James, 67, 71
Coren, Stanley, 112
Cortisol
    function, 20, 22
    levels, 32
Cretinism, 33

**D**
*Dateline,* 240
Delivery systems, 134–135
Dentali, Steven, 83–84, 91, 152
Depression
    sleep and, 126
    St. John's wort, 156–157
Dermopathy, 149–150
Desyrel, 57
Diana, Princess of Wales, 247
Diet
    American, 171–172
    guidelines, 186–187
Dietary Supplement Health and Edu-
    cation Act of 1994
    FDA and, 231, 235–240
    terms of, 238–239
Dihydrokavain, 85
Dioscorides, 230
Dopamine, 153–154
Dosage
    kava, 133–136
    St. John's wort, 158
Dossey, Dr. Larry, 203
Driving
    accidents, 112
    kava use and, 145–146
Drugs
    hard *vs.* soft, 211–213
    interactions, 142–145
Drummond, Edward, 58
DSHEA, *see* Dietary Supplement Health
    and Education Act of 1994
Dystonia, 154

**E**
Economics
    agriculture, 217–220, 225–226
    herbal medicine, 229–231
    kava, 241
Edison, Thomas, 113
EEG, *see* Electroencephalograph
Effexor, 57
Eidelson, Judy, 23
Elderly
    benzodiazepines and, 122
    statistics, 124
    ginkgo biloba aids, 165–166
    insomnia, 103–104
    sleep and, 119–120
Electroencephalograph, 116
Electromyogram, 116
Electro-oculogram, 116
Ellis, Cynthia, 167
Ellis, William, 72
EMDR, *see* Eye movement desensitization and reprocessing
EMG, *see* Electromyogram
Endorphins, 31–33
EOG, *see* Electro-oculogram
EPS, *see* Extrapyramidal symptoms
ESCOP, *see* The European Scientific Cooperative for Phytomedicines
Essential fatty acids, 178
Ethnopharmacological Search for Psychoactive Drugs Symposium, 210, 212
Europe, *see also* Specific countries
    herbal medicine
        economics, 229–231
        popularity, 93–95
European Scientific Cooperative for Phytomedicines, 231
Exercise, 200
Exhaustion, 22
Extraction process, 82
Extrapyramidal symptoms, 154
Eye movement desensitization and reprocessing, 45, 47

**F**
Farmers' Rights, 225
Fatigue, 181
Fats, 185–186
Faust, Dr. Robert, 223
FDA, *see* Food and Drug Administration
Fight-or-flight syndrome, 4, 14
Fiji, 220–222
Flex-Herb, 166
Folic acid, 174–175

Food and Drug Administration
    clinical trials, 234–235
    Commission E *vs.*, 94, 231
    DSHEA, 235–240
    herbal medicine regulation, 233–235
    kava regulation, 240
Forster, Johann Georg, 71
Freedman, Daniel X., 212
Friedman, Gary, 108–109, 208, 221
Fungicides, 110
fX Rush, 146

**G**
GABA, *see* Gamma-aminobutyric acid
Gajdusek, Carleton, 210
Galen, 171
Gamma-aminobutyric acid, 87–88
Garner, 150
GAS, *see* General adaptation syndrome
General adaptation syndrome, 21
Genes
    anxiety and, 41–42
    engineering, 223–225
Germany
    Commission E monograph, 94–95
    herb use, 93–94
    kava use, 7
Ginger, 166
Ginkgo biloba, 165
Ginseng, 163–164
Gittleman, Ann Louise, 105
Glucose, 125
Gordon, Barbara, 63
Gratitude, 201–203
Green tea, 189
Gruenwald, Joerg, 95
Gunn, William, 151
Guppy study, 32–33

**H**
Habituation, 151
Halpren, Steven, 197
Hammarskjold, 205
*The Happy Isle of Oceania,* 68
Harrisson, Tom, 9, 208
Hartman & Newhart, 233
Hawaii
    agriculture, 222–223
    kava ceremony, 1–4
    kava use, 79
Health care, 245
Herbal Ecstasy, 240
Herbal medicine
    consumption, 233
    statistics, 237–238

Herbal medicine *(continued)*
  insomnia, 159–162
  kava mixtures, 155–159, 166–168
  market growth, 229–233
  misuse, 239–240
  pharmaceuticals *vs.*, 233–235
History, 70–73
Hoffer, Dr. Abram, 37
Hoffmann, David, 248
Holmes, T., 15
Hops, 161
Huxley, Aldous, 211
5-Hydroxytryptophan, 130, 179
Hypoglycemia
  description, 180–186
  diet, 188
Hypothalamus, 20, 22

**I**

*I'm Dancing As Fast As I Can,* 63
Immune system, 22
Inner player, 48–49
Inositol, 174
Insomnia, *see also* Sleep
  categories, 118
  causes, 118
  contributing factors, 119
  elderly and, 103–104
  herbal remedies, 159–162
  incidence, 102, 117–118
  origins, 118–119
  treatment, 61
  treatments, 118
Instant powdered extract, 137
Intellectual property rights,
    226–227
Iron, 176–177
Irwin, Dr. Michael, 113

**J**

John Paul II, 76
Johnson, Lyndon, 76

**K**

Kabat-Zinn, Jon, 195
Kava, *see also* Kavalactones
  active ingredients, 82–85
  adaptogens with, 162–166
  addiction, 151–152
    aborigine case, 152
  alcohol interactions, 145
  alcohol *vs.*, 77
  analgesic effects, 88–90, 101–102
  anticonvulsant effects, 88–90,
    101–102
  antifungal effects, 110

anxiety, 86–87
  clinical studies, 96–101
bars, 79–80
benzodiazepines *vs.*, 99–100
bladder infections, 110
botany, 69–70
ceremony
  decline, 78–79
  description, 1–4
  Samoan, 75
CFS, 107
children and, 105–106
commission E monographs
  effectiveness study, 96–97
  safety study, 141–142
  side effects, 147–148
components, 84–85
conflict resolution, 207–209
in context, 206–207
contraindications, 142
council, 240–241
cultivation
  economics, 217–220, 225–226
  Fiji, 220–222
  Hawaii, 222–223
  obstacles, 218–220
  opportunities, 218–220
  Vanuatu, 220–222
delivery systems, 134–135
dermopathy, 149–150
dopamine interaction, 153–154
dosage, 133–137
drug interactions, 142–145
economics, 241
effects, 69
empowerment, 76
European use, 7
experiencing, 214–215
extraction process, 82
FDA and, 240
food with, 139
forms, 137–138
fresh experience, 210–211
function, 91–92
GABA and, 87–88
habituation, 151
herbal combinations, 155–159,
    166–168
history, 1, 68, 70–73
industry, ethics, 249
local anesthesia, 107–108
menopause, 104–105
message, 205–206
modern use, 79–80
muscle relaxation, 88–90
nervous system, 86

nicotine withdrawal, 188
with other herbs, 9
overview, 243
placebo effect, 67–68, 97–99
for pleasure, 211–212
preparation, 71, 76–77
products, 138–139
properties, 81–82
quality of life and, 249–250
safety, 141–142, 147
sex and, 209–210
sleep and, 127–128
St. John's wort with, 158–159
stress and, 215–216, 244–245
taste, 68
tolerance, 137, 151
traditional uses, 72–73, 108–109
use
   duration, 139, 142
   responsible, 144–145
uses, 106–107
visual effects, 150
withdrawal, 151
*Kava: The Pacific Elixir,* 108
Kavain, 85, 89
Kavalactones, *see also* Kava
content, 136
properties, 73
standardization, 84–85
synthesized, 83
Kilham, Chris, 80
Kline, Nathan, 212
Klinger, 150
Konanui, Jerry, 223
Kripke, Dr. Daniel, 129

**L**
Lader, Malcolm, 64
*Lancet,* 212, 232
Learning, 125–126
Lebot, Vincent, 108, 127, 152,
   219–220
Lemert, E. M., 210
Levine, Andy, 138
Levine, Peter, 42
Licorice, 164
Lifestyles
American, 191–194
being in present, 198–200
nature, 248–249
quality, 249–250
sleep and, 130–131
Lindstrom, Lamont, 152
Local anesthesia, 107–108
Los Angeles Police Department,
   146

**M**
Macronutrients, 179–180, 185–186
Magnesium, 177
Marijuana, 212–213
*Markings,* 205
Meat, red, 186
*Medical Herbalism,* 91
*Medicine Hunting in Paradise,* 80
Meditation, 195, 201
Melatonin, 129–130
*The Melatonin Miracle,* 129
Memory, 125–126
Menopause, 104–105
Mental health
amino acids, 178–179
cutbacks, 64
fatty acids, 178
macronutrients, 179–180,
   185–186
minerals and, 175–177
pharmaceutical industry, 63–65
vitamins and, 172–175
Merlin, Mark, 152
Milk thistle, 188
Mind-body continuum
description, 33–38
research, 38–39
Mindfulness, 195
Minerals, 175–177
*Molecules of Emotion,* 87
Monkey mind, 195
Monoamine oxidase, 30
Monoamine oxidase inhibitors, 55
Morrison, James, 102
Mortality, 127–129
Moyers, Bill, 246
Muscle relaxing, 88–90, 101–102
Mushrooms, reishi, 164–165
Music, 196–198

**N**
Nakamals, 79–80, 138
Naranjo, Claudio, 212
National Sleep Foundation, 114,
   118–119
*The Natural Mind,* 214
*Natural Products Quarterly Review,* 231
Nature, 196–198
Nervous system, 86–87
Neurofeedback, 201
Neurons, 29–30
Neurotransmitters
definition, 30–31
restoration, 126
*New England Journal of Medicine,* 8
New Hope, 233

*Newsweek,* 6, 11
Niacin, 174
Nicholson, Jack, 25
Nicotine, 187
Niebuhr, Rheinhold, 200
Nike, 113
NSF, *see* National Sleep Foundation

**O**
Oat seeds, 166
Obessive-compulsive disorder, 25
Optimism, 201–203
Orthomolecular, 37
Osmond, Dr. Humphrey, 37
*Overcoming Anxiety without Tranquilizers,* 59, 62

**P**
Pacific Islanders, 102
Pantothenic acid, 174
Parkinson's disease, 153–154
Passion flower, 161–162
Pauling, Linus, 37
Paxil, 56
Pellagra, 36
Pert, Candace, 87
PET, *see* Positron emission tomography
Pfeiffer, Carl, 212
Pharmaceutical industry
    herbal medicine, 233–235
    sleep aids, 63–65
Phobias, 24
Phosphatidylserine, 179
Phytomedicines, 93
Pierpaoli, Dr. Walter, 129
Pituitary gland, 20, 22
Placebo effect, 67–68, 97–99
Polling Company survey, 192
Popky, A. J., 188
Positron emission tomography, 125
Post-traumatic stress disorder, 43–44
Potassium, 176
Powdered kava root, 137–138
Prayer, 203
Prisoners, 208
Processed foods, 186
Progressive relaxation, 200–201
Proteins, 185
Prozac
    description, 55–56
    pediatric, 106
Psychotherapy, 6
PTSD, *see* Post-traumatic stress disorder

Pyridoxine, 174
Pythagoras, 200

**R**
Rahe, R., 15
Ram Dass, 199–200
Rapid eye movement
    importance, 125–127
    sleep occurrence, 116–117
RAS, *see* Reticular activation system
Ravuvu, Asesela, 76
RDA, *see* Recommended daily allowance
Recommended daily allowance, 173
Red meat, 186
Reishi mushrooms, 164–165
Relaxation, progressive, 200–201
REM, *see* Rapid eye movement
Resistance reaction, 21–22
Reticular activation system, 115
Riboflavin, 174
Riegleson, Dr. William, 129
Rifkin, Jeremy, 223
Ritalin, 106
Roth, Dr. Thomas, 112
Russia, 163

**S**
Samoan legend, 73–74
*Savage Civilization,* 9, 208
Schultes, Richard, 212
Self-awareness, 194–195
Selye, Dr. Hans, 17, 19–21, 23
Serenity Prayer, 200
Serotonin
    definition, 30
    function, 56
    health effects, 32
    sleep and, 130
Serotonin re-uptake inhibitors, 55–56
Service, 201–203
Serzone, 57
Sex, 209–210
Shulgin, Alexander, 212
Siegel, Dr. Ron, 213
Silverman, Wayne, 95
Singh, Nirbhay, 167
Singh, Y. N., 88–89, 101–102
Skin rash, 149–150
Skullcap, 166
Sleep, *see also* Insomnia
    age and, 119–120
    depression and, 126
    habits, 114–115
    hygiene, 131

immune system and, 113–114
importance, 111–113
kava
    dosage, 136–137
kava and, 127–128
latency, 116
learning and, 125–126
logs, 131
loss, effects, 112
memory and, 125–126
promoting behavior, 130–131
REM, 116–117
serotonin and, 130
spindles, 116
stages, 115–117
work and, 113–114
Sleep aids, *see also* Benzodiazepines
mortality, 127–129
natural, 129–130
recommended use, 120–121
Smith, Ed, 159, 166, 221, 222
Smoking, 187–188
Social Readjustment Rating Scale,
    15–17
Sodium, 176
Soft drinks, 186–187
South Pacific, 73–77, 226, *see also*
    Specific countries
Spirituality, 203
St. John's wort
    characteristics, 156–158
    dosage, 158
    European sales, 230
    kava with, 158–159
    popularity, 6–7
    sleep and, 130
    synthesized, 83
    tyramine effect, 157
Standardization
    dosage, 135–136
    kavalactones, 84–85
Stone, Dr. Hal, 52
Stone, Dr. Sidra, 52
Stress
    addiction, 5
    awareness and, 194–195
    case studies, 49–52
    costs, 4–5
    definition, 14
    exercise and, 200
    function, 21
    health effects, 33–34
    hypoglycemia and, 180–186
    immune system and, 22
    incidence, 4

inner voice, 48–49
kava combinations, 167–168
kava for, 215–216, 244–245
lifestyles and, 193–194
management, 196–203
    principles, 198–199
    tips, 202
mind-body continuum, 33–38
modern, 12–13
overcoming, 27–28
phases, 21–23
physical effects, 18–19
physiology, 20–23
prehistoric, 11–12
response, 17–20
risk assessment, 14–17
survival, 13–14
treatments
    conventional, 5–6
    natural, 6–7
triggers, 25–27
vitamins and, 172–175
Synapses, 30

**T**
Tagaloa Ui, 74–75
*Talking Back to Prozac*, 62
Theroux, Paul, 68
Thiamin, 173
Tolerance
    benzodiazepines, 123–125
    kava, 137, 151
Traditional resources rights, 227
Trauma, 42–43
Tricyclics, 54–55
Tryptophan
    availablity, 179
    regulation, 234
    L-Tryptophan, 130
*20/20*, 6
Tylenol, 234

**U**
United States, *see* Americans

**V**
Valerian, 159–160, 188
Vanuatu, 220–222
Van Veen, A. G., 82, 107
Violence, cycle, 208
Vision, 150
Vitamin B complex, 173–175
Vitamin C
    properties, 175
    smoking and, 187

Vitamins, 172–175
Voice dialogue, 49–52
Volz, H.P., 97–99, 142

**W**
*Waking the Tiger Within,* 42
Wasson, Gordon, 212
Water, chlorinated, 187
Weil, Andrew, 214
Wellbutrin, 57
Whole grains, 186
Willard, Terry, 69, 101, 110, 166, 207
Withdrawal, 151

Work
   hours spent, 192
   sleep and, 113–114
World Health Organization, 232
Wright, Dr. Jonathan, 164

**X**
Xanax, 143–144

**Z**
Zinc, 177
Zoloft, 56